Supporting People with Learning Disabilities in

HEALTH & SOCIAL CARE

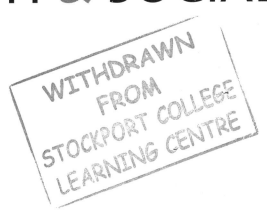

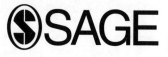

Supporting People with Learning Disabilities in

HEALTH & SOCIAL CARE

Edited by
Eric Broussine & Kim Scarborough

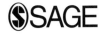

Los Angeles | London | New Delhi
Singapore | Washington DC

First published 2012

SAGE Publications Ltd
1 Oliver's Yard
55 City Road
London EC1Y 1SP

SAGE Publications Inc.
2455 Teller Road
Thousand Oaks, California 91320

SAGE Publications India Pvt Ltd
B 1/I 1 Mohan Cooperative Industrial Area
Mathura Road
New Delhi 110 044

SAGE Publications Asia-Pacific Pte Ltd
3 Church Street
#10-04 Samsung Hub
Singapore 049483

Library of Congress Control Number: 2011928955

British Library Cataloguing in Publication data

A catalogue record for this book is available from the British Library

ISBN 978-1-84920-083-7
ISBN 978-1-84920-084-4 (pbk)

Typeset by C&M Digitals (P) Ltd, Chennai, India
Printed by MPG Books Group, Bodmin, Cornwall
Printed on paper from sustainable resources

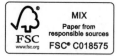

MIX
Paper from
responsible sources
FSC
www.fsc.org FSC® C018575

CONTENTS

LIST OF FIGURES AND TABLES

FIGURES

TABLES

NOTES ON THE EDITORS AND CONTRIBUTORS

Eric Broussine is a Senior Lecturer at the University of the West of England, Bristol. He teaches a range of subjects across all nursing programmes but specifically focuses on communication and interpersonal skills. He has a particular interest in the mental health needs of people with learning disabilities and autism. He chairs a nurse elective group and has developed strong links with learning disability services in Croatia.

Kim Scarborough is a National Teaching Fellow who works at the University of the West of England, Bristol. She has worked with people who have a learning disability for 30 years and now focuses on their involvement in the education of health and social care professionals.

Jonathan Coles is a Senior Lecturer in learning disabilities studies in the Faculty of Health and Life Sciences at the University of the West of England. He has both a practice and research interest in the involvement of service users and carers in both social care service development and also education and training for social care staff.

Jackie Edwards is the mother of 3 young men. Her middle son has learning disabilities. Jackie has worked with family carers since 1997 highlighting the need for professionals and families to work in partnership to ensure the best outcomes for individuals who are not able to speak for themselves.

Sue Hogarth works for Gloucestershire County Council as the Learning Disability Partnership Board Support Officer. Sue has worked for over 20 years in the learning disability field, including the development and management of courses in further education. Sue has also set up and supported members to run an independent self-advocacy group.

Dawn Rooke is a mother to three boys, two of which have autistic spectrum disorders and learning difficulties, and carer to a husband with complex medical conditions.

Dawn volunteers as a trainer in Transition, Person Centred Thinking Skills and is also a Visiting Lecturer at UWE in Bristol, where she speaks on autism, person centred planning and the carer's views and experiences.

Neil Summers is a Senior Lecturer working at The University of the West of England, Bristol. He has been working with children with special educational needs and their families for 30 years. He has a research interest in how professionals support families with children with special needs. He has experience of facilitating mixed groups of professionals, students, carers and users of services. His work is focussed on collaboration and partnership with families and has an interest in widening access in higher education.

Robert Parode is Programme Leader for the BSc (Hons) Learning Disabilities Nursing programme at UWE Bristol. Robert also teaches a range of modules related to communication, relationship building, inter-professional working and challenging behaviour. He has been a Registered Nurse for 25 years, a Senior Lecturer for 19 years and a Social Worker for 10 years.

Matthew Godsell is a Senior Lecturer in the School of Learning Disabilities in the Faculty of Health and Life Sciences at the University of the West of England, Bristol. His current interests are social policy, developing evidence based practice and the history of specialised services for people with learning disabilities.

Amelia Oughtibridge has a background in both community residential services and community nursing for people with learning disabilities. She has specialist expertise in meeting the complex health care needs of the population, in particular end of life care, and is the current Vice Chair of the Palliative Care for People with Learning Disabilities (PCPLD) Network. As Lead Nurse and Team Co-ordinator for Wiltshire Learning Disability Services, Amelia continues to develop her interest in health facilitation and promotion.

Alan Nuttall has worked as a nurse for people with learning disabilities for over 30 years, as a ward and residential home manager. He has been involved in creating several new residential services for people with complex emotional needs. He is currently employed as Positive Behaviour Support Manager for Milestones Trust, an organisation which supports people with learning disabilities and mental health needs, including dementia.

Wendy Goodman is a registered mental health nurse with 22 years' post registration experience working in forensic health care including 12 years in medium secure provision and 10 years as senior nurse with a community forensic learning disabilities team. Her current role involves providing assessment and therapeutic interventions for offenders who have learning disabilities in community settings.

Sarah Campbell has 27 years experience as a nurse and 12 years working in forensic and offending healthcare in the Gloucester area. In 2007 Sarah returned to offender health, taking the role of Mental Health Service

Manager and then Clinical Services Manager at HMP Gloucester. She is currently the Service Manager for Mental Health at HMP Hewell in Redditch.

Crispin Hebron is a Non Medical Consultant in a Mental Health and Learning Disability Foundation Trust. He has previously worked in the NHS and third sector in a range of nursing, project and management roles. He is currently contributing as an investigator to the Confidential Inquiry into premature deaths in people with learning disabilities run by the Norah Fry Research Centre at Bristol University.

INTRODUCTION

Eric Broussine and Kim Scarborough

RATIONALE FOR THE BOOK

Over the last ten years there has been growing concern over the treatment of people who have a learning disability when they require healthcare interventions (Department of Health, 2001; Mencap, 2004; Disabilities Rights Commission, 2006; Mencap, 2007; Abraham, 2009). Partnership working between health and social care providers and families is often seen as poor with resulting negative consequences for the people who have learning disabilities (Michael Report, 2008). Also, strategy papers have been produced that seek to redress the inequalities that people with learning disabilities face (The Scottish Government, 2000; Northern Ireland Executive, 2005; Welsh Assembly Government, 2007; Department of Health, 2009). A common theme in these reports and papers is the need to treat people with learning disabilities equitably, to use person centred approaches and to work in effective partnerships with people with learning disabilities, their families, paid carers and the wide range of health and social care professionals and others who are involved in people's lives.

The Michael Report (2008) specifically highlights that health and social care staff need better training in how to support people with learning disabilities. One of the Report's recommendations is that services need to make reasonable adjustments, which is about ensuring that services demonstrate flexibility, inclusivity and partnership working when supporting and treating people with learning disabilities. However, understanding what reasonable adjustment looks like is an important factor in ensuring it happens. This book has been written to support people employed in health and social care services to respond to the need for improvements in how professionals provide services to people with learning disabilities and how they can make reasonable adjustment in their practice. The book is designed to encourage the reader to review their knowledge and skills and to develop strategies to improve their practice, in order to promote inclusion and positive outcomes for people who have a learning disability.

A WORD ABOUT WORDS

In this book we use the term 'learning disabilities' as this is the language used in UK health policy and by organisations such as Mencap. However, we acknowledge that there is controversy around the use of terminology. Some, but by no means all, user-led groups prefer the term 'learning difficulty' as they feel it represents a social model of care (see Chapter 2) and there is a gradual swing towards the use of the term 'intellectual disability' or 'intellectual impairment'. Our thoughts are that we are talking about people and any of the labels above will be both supported and challenged; what is important is the need to see past these labels to the people we are serving. Many terms used historically to label people with learning disabilities are now derogatory, insulting and degrading. The language used suppressed people and reinforced their disability, focussing on what they could not do rather than on their strengths, abilities and potential. The abusive language associated with learning disability continues to be used without thought in playgrounds, workplaces and public services or, more menacingly, used with thought to degrade, frighten and oppress people. What matters is how you consider your use of language and how you act towards people. How do you show respect, how do you display that you value the individual and demonstrate that they are worthy and equal citizens? In this book, we want to engender a belief in equality and the human value of people with learning disabilities by helping you understand what living with a learning disability means, and how your actions display your values and attitudes. We ask you to be mindful of the language you use, try to reflect the language that individuals themselves use but most importantly act in a way that demonstrates your positive regard for people who may have a learning disability, ensuring the person is – first and foremost – a cared about and cared for individual.

We recognise that 'learning disabilities' is a convenient term which describes an extremely diverse and heterogeneous group of the UK population. In the course of the book, the chapter authors refer to people with learning disabilities throughout the life cycle, to those with mild to moderate learning disabilities through to severe and profound learning disabilities, including those with physical and sensory impairments, people on the autistic spectrum and those with associated health needs. In addition people with learning disabilities live in a variety of settings, access a range of statutory, voluntary and independent service provisions and engage in a wide range of educational, leisure and work activities. The diversity of this group therefore acknowledges that working and forming relationships must be based on a person centred, individualised approach.

AIMS AND THEMES

The principle aim of this book is to bring the reader up to date with contemporary practice in working and forming positive relationships with people with learning disabilities across the UK. The book explores twenty-first century practice encompassing formal and informal policy, the complex power dynamics within relationships and current philosophy, and the values of inclusion, rights, choices, independence and being in control (Department of Health [DH], 2001). The initial chapters concentrate on themes of empowerment, vulnerability, the medical and social model of care, citizenship, self-advocacy and the personalisation agenda, presenting different views of person centred planning and relationships between people with learning disabilities, families and professionals. Two chapters carefully consider relationships and effective communication. Later chapters explore what evidence based care is and the specific evidence based practice for some contemporary issues for people with learning disabilities – including mental and physical health issues – and the inclusion of people with learning disabilities in the criminal justice system. The book concludes with a review of professional practice which includes codes of conduct, person centred care and ethics.

The chapter authors come from a variety of backgrounds, including parents of young people with learning disabilities, health professionals who specialise in learning disabilities practice and learning disabilities nurse lecturers. We have found that authors from different backgrounds emphasise different aspects of living with a learning disability and view this as a strength of the book.

THE CHAPTERS

Chapter 1　Social Policy Tensions – Empowerment and Vulnerability

Chapter 1 explores twentieth and twenty-first century attitudes and associated social policy towards people with learning disabilities. It highlights contradictory evidence which suggests that people labelled with a learning disability want to be empowered and take more control over their own lives. However, at the same time they are seen as vulnerable and at risk of abuse and exploitation, and therefore in need of protection. The chapter addresses these tensions in social policy by discussing formal and informal legislation and research. Chapter 1 concludes by recommending that health and social care staff need to be vigilant with regard to these conflicting values and work to empower people while recognising their potential vulnerabilities.

Chapter 2　The History and Context of Learning Disability: A Parent's Perspective

This chapter presents a parent's perspective of cultural and policy changes over the last forty years. It outlines the medical and social model of disability, and the impact these models have on individuals with a learning disability and their families. It further examines the concept of inclusive practice which, it is argued, places more emphasis on the role of families to care and provide for their family member. This can raise anxieties as responsibility shifts from services to the family. Chapter 2 also offers a critical view of Person Centred Planning (PCP) and the personalisation agenda, and argues that parents and families living with change to policy and culture are often left feeling confused and disorientated. The chapter concludes by suggesting that policy and culture is constantly evolving.

Chapter 3　Enabling People with Learning Disabilities to be Valued Citizens

The emphasis of this chapter is about promoting citizenship and self-advocacy for people with learning disabilities. It explores the notion that through a process of empowerment people are more able and willing to become active participants in their community and influence changes in practice. An example is offered where people with learning disabilities contributed to national policy about hate crime towards people with disabilities. Barriers to effective citizenship – particularly for those with specific complex needs and from black and ethnic minorities – are also highlighted. The chapter emphasises the contribution of person centred approaches and planning to citizenship and also the importance of employment for people with learning disabilities.

Chapter 4   Living with a Learning Disability

Chapter 4 illuminates a range of formal and informal support mechanisms that are available to people with learning disabilities and their families through the life continuum to enable them to live a full life. Illustrated with real life stories, the chapter highlights a range of concerns about and solutions to accessing an ordinary life at each stage of a person's development and the effects on their families. Pre-school, school, transition from children to adult services, adult education, occupation and work, leisure and social life, and the needs of older people are all explored with examples of good practice and positive solutions.

Chapter 5   Enabling Families: A Model of Helping

The author examines a range of empirical evidence which supported a pathological and, therefore, negative perspective of parents' experiences of caring for a child with a learning disability. Quality of help to parents was often poor, resulting in deterioration in the relationship between parents and services. An alternative model of helping is offered based in empowerment and partnership working. Chapter 5 investigates the complex dynamics of families asking for and receiving help from services, and the consequences of both negative and positive worker qualities on parent–worker relationships. The chapter suggests that parents value a consistent relationship and that they prefer a socially skilled and/or emotionally intelligent worker rather than a worker providing only instrumental support.

Chapter 6   Building Positive Relationships with People with Learning Disabilities

This chapter investigates the skills and qualities necessary in promoting positive, therapeutic relationships with people with learning disabilities. Rogers' (1957) three core conditions of empathy, congruence and unconditional positive regard are outlined, as are Egan's (2007) micro-skills of listening and attending. Some challenges of active listening with people with specific needs are highlighted. The chapter examines the concepts of self-awareness, by introducing the Johari Window (Luft 1969), 'the therapeutic use of self' and reflective practice and argues how these ideas contribute to a better understanding of ourselves and, ultimately, has a positive impact on the self-esteem of clients and the carer–client relationship.

Chapter 7   Promoting Effective Communication

This chapter appraises the importance of communication and emphasises a range of understanding and expression barriers that people with learning disabilities experience. A Total Communication model is introduced that provides a framework for the chapter. Pragmatic strategies are provided for the reader to address some of these communication difficulties, including scenarios to help illustrate points made. Alternative and Augmentative Communication techniques are briefly described, including the use of Intensive Interaction, Makaton and other signing systems. A hierarchy of communication strategies is provided, along with how to access further information and advice about specific approaches.

Chapter 8   Health and Well-being

Strategies to promote collaborative practice between specialist services for people with learning disabilities and generic healthcare services are discussed in this chapter. The benefits of Patient Passports for hospital staff – and what they contain – are described. A multitude of health risks and social determinants which disadvantage people are also examined. The Michael Report (2008) also identifies a range of health inequalities including diagnostic overshadowing and communication difficulties. Two models of evidence based practice are introduced to encourage stronger links between theory and practice. Chapter 8 provides two case studies which facilitate a better understanding of how Person Centred Planning and evidence based practice enhance the well-being of people with learning disabilities.

Chapter 9   Epilepsy, Pain and End of Life Care: Healthcare Issues for People with Learning Disabilities

The author of Chapter 9 explores the assessment of complex health needs, taking into account a person's history, their mental capacity, their vulnerability and risk factors when admitted into hospital and the need to assess their optimum health. Epilepsy assessment and management is examined, including medication control. The risks of people with learning disabilities in pain and the difficulties of assessing levels of pain are highlighted. A model for using analgesia for pain is advocated and a pain management tool is introduced. End of life care is addressed with recommendations that partnership working between the individual, their family, other carers, GPs, medical specialists and palliative care services is regarded as best practice.

Chapter 10   Meeting some Specific Mental Health Needs of People with Learning Disabilities

Chapter 10 explores some general principles around the diagnosis and assessment of mental ill health, medication treatments and psychological interventions. Mental Health law, with particular emphasis on the Mental Capacity Act (2005), is also discussed. The chapter's author argues that there exist some perceived tensions between specialist learning disability and generic mental health services and that these pressures impact on the quality of services delivered. Two specific mental health problems – drug and alcohol abuse and dementia – are addressed as a means of illustrating the application of the promoted values. The chapter offers 'real stories' to further supplement context and meaning.

Chapter 11   People with Learning Disabilities in the Criminal Justice System

This chapter takes the reader on a journey of what it might be like for someone with a learning disability to go through the Criminal Justice System (CJS). It begins with a brief outline of the number of people with learning disabilities in the CJS, followed by first contact with the police and the role of the appropriate adult. Courts, sentencing and court liaison including court assessment and referral service are considered. Probation and community orders are also explored, along with the introduction of two therapeutic community programmes. Screening for a learning disability, making information accessible and promoting prison in-reach teams are all approaches used to improve prison healthcare. Finally, Chapter 11 discusses positive outcomes and leaving prison. A theme of the chapter is the need for a wide range of services to liaise effectively with each other and encourage learning disability awareness training.

Chapter 12   Professional Practice

The final chapter scrutinises factors and complexities of professional practice in the context of working with people with learning disabilities. Professionalism is defined and a social model of disability is advocated as an appropriate approach to delivering professional practice. Aims of professional conduct are highlighted – such as promoting inclusive practice, ensuring positive outcomes and enhancing quality of life – as well as making reasonable adjustment. Six common themes within codes of conduct across disciplines are examined as well as discussing the value of networking to improve the lives of people. Accessing appropriate services and assessment are used to illuminate best professional practice. Chapter 12 concludes by articulating the need for practitioners to become more collaborative in making judgements and in clinical decision making with the emphasis being on consent, ethics and confidentiality.

USING THIS BOOK TO IMPROVE YOUR PRACTICE

Reflection points

Reflection points are a key component of the structure of this book and appear throughout. A primary objective of the reflection points within each chapter is to help you apply your reading to your own practice. By reading each chapter, completing the reflective questions and considering the scenarios, you will be able to build a picture of the strengths, needs, opportunities and threats of and to your practice. You can then consider what areas of your knowledge, skills and values you are pleased with and will want to maintain and which areas you are unsure about and may need to develop further. Record the areas of your personal and professional practice that you can improve as a result of your reading and reflecting; also note what areas need enhancing and clearly state what you need to change, what you need to learn, and how this will improve your practice. The outcome is that you will have developed a clear idea of your practice in relation to people with learning disabilities. This book, therefore, has a pragmatic dimension and is designed to help you build stronger links between learning disability contemporary theory and real life, in an increasingly complex and busy health and social care environment.

Action-planning

Once you have identified key action points resulting from the consolidation of your learning, you will be in a position to develop an action plan to improve your practice. You should select practice changes that are within your sphere of authority for them to be achievable. You may wish to consider the action plan in relation to your specific role and responsibilities, or extend this to your team's role, or consider possible changes at organisational level. The aim of action planning is to support you in taking appropriate actions that are commensurate with your caring, clinical or management responsibilities.

To start action planning you might want to come up with a list of Tiny Achievable Tickable Targets – TATTs (Mosley, 1996). These list what you want to achieve and as you complete them you can 'tick them off'. It can be satisfying knowing that you are contributing to, safeguarding and promoting 'reasonable adjustments' that improve the lives of people with learning disabilities in your service.

SMART objectives

To achieve your targets it can be useful to think carefully about what you are going to do. SMART objectives are a constructive way of establishing an action plan that can be monitored and evaluated. The term is an acronym that means:

- **S**pecific – Objectives should specify what they want to achieve. For example, what are you going to do, what do you need to focus on, are you precise enough?
- **M**easurable – You should be able to measure whether you are meeting the objectives or not. Consider ways of measuring your objectives.
- **A**chievable – Are the objectives you set achievable and attainable? Can they be achieved within the context and realities of practice?
- **R**ealistic – Can you realistically achieve the objectives with the resources you have?
- **T**ime – When do you want to achieve the set objectives? Is your time frame short term (over the next few days or weeks) or long term (over the next few months?) (Doran, 1981)

Using SMART objectives will encourage you to organise your thoughts and give you a clear sense of direction for your learning. By following this simple acronym, you will be in control and proactive about what can be achieved within the timescales that you establish. Do not try to set yourself too many SMART goals at once, take one tickable target at a time and plan how you are going to achieve it by setting a SMART objective.

Some reflection points present opportunities for you to consider your own practice. Structured reflection can enhance your learning. Driscoll's What? So What? Now What? model (Figure 1) of structured reflection (Driscoll, 2007) can be used as a tool to give the reflective points deeper meaning or to reflect on the outcomes of your SMART objectives. The model has a series of questions to ask yourself (Figure 2), but the idea is for you to use this model as a framework and not to stick rigidly to the questions it poses, as this may stifle your own curiosity about a situation and direction of approach.

Coupled with the range of reflective points within the book you should be able to identify the areas of your practice that are inclusive, highlighting your strengths and gifts. It will also help you to identify areas of your practice which could be improved. Alternatively, you may wish to use an exercise

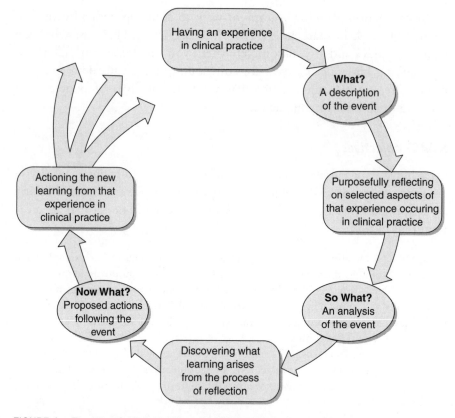

FIGURE 1   *The What? Model of Structured Reflection and its Relationship to an Experiential Learning Cycle*

Source: Figures 1 and 2 are reproduced with kind permission of John Driscoll (2007: 44–5).

as a stepping stone to doing some further research or to find additional information about a situation you have experienced. The outcomes of participating in the reflection points, developing tickable targets, using the SMART objectives alongside Driscoll's (2007) structured model of reflection are to gain deeper insights into you, your team and your organisation's approach to working and forming positive relationships with people with learning disabilities in health and social care practice.

We hope that by using the activities in this book you can develop your practice and in so doing begin to make a positive impact, through your learning and contributions, to the lives of people with learning disabilities. We hope that in reading this book you will not be passive but rather an active learner, inspired to influence and make real changes to your practice. People with learning disabilities are not asking for much, they simply want to be treated the same as you and me and to be valued as

1 A *description* of the event

What? trigger questions:

- is the purpose of returning to this situation?
- happened?
- did I see/do?
- was my reaction to it?
- did other people do who were involved in this?

2 An *analysis* of the event

So What? trigger questions:

- How did I feel at the time of the event?
- Were those feelings I had any different from those of other people who were also involved at the time?
- Are my feelings now, after the event, any different from what I experienced at the time?
- Do I still feel troubled, if so, in what way?
- What were the effects of what I did (or did not do)?
- What positive aspects now emerge for me from the event that happened in practice?
- What have I noticed about my behaviour in practice by taking a more measured look at it?
- What observations does any person helping me to reflect on my practice make of the way I acted at the time?

3 Proposed *actions* following the event

Now What? trigger questions:

- What are the implications for me and others in clinical practice based on what I have described and analysed?
- What difference does it make if I choose to do nothing?
- Where can I get more information to face a similar situation again?
- How can I modify my practice if a similar situation was to happen again?
- What help do I need to help me 'action' the results of my reflections?
- Which aspect should be tackled first?
- How will I notice that I am any different in clinical practice?
- What is the main learning that I take from reflecting on my practice in this way?

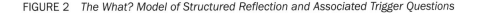

FIGURE 2   *The What? Model of Structured Reflection and Associated Trigger Questions*

human beings – to be treated fairly, with equality of access to health and social care services and the health outcomes that all members of society have come to expect.

REFERENCES

Abraham, A. (2009) *Six Lives: The Provision of Public Services to People with Learning Disabilities. Part One: Overview and Summary Investigation Reports.* London: Local Government Ombudsman. [online] Available from http://www.ombudsman.org.uk/__data/assets/pdf_file/0013/1408/six-lives-part1-overview.pdf, accessed 03.09.2010.

Department of Health (2001) *Valuing People: A New Strategy for Learning Disability for the 21st century.* London: Department of Health.

Department of Health (2009) *Valuing People Now – A New Three Year Strategy for People with Learning Disabilities.* London: Department of Health.

Disability Rights Commission (2006) *Equal Treatment: Closing the Gap. A Formal Investigation into Physical Health Inequalities Experienced by People with Learning Disabilities and/or Mental Health Problems.* [online] Available from: http://83.137.212.42/sitearchive/DRC/library/health_investigation.html#Finalreportsandsummaries, accessed 02.03.10.

Doran, G.T. (1981) 'There's a S.M.A.R.T. way to write management's goals and objectives', *Management Review*, 70 (11): 35–6.

Driscoll, J. (2007) *Practising Clinical Supervision. A Reflective Approach for Healthcare Professionals* (2nd edn). London, BailliereTindall.

Egan, G. (2007) *The Skilled Helper: A Problem–Management and Opportunity–Development approach to helping* (8th edn). Belmont, CA: Thomson Brooks/Cole.

Luft, J. (1969) *On Human Interaction.* Palo Alto, CA: National Press.

Mencap (2004) *Treat Me Right: Better Healthcare for People with a Learning Disability.* London: Mencap.

Mencap (2007) *Death by Indifference.* London: Mencap.

Mental Capacity Act (2005). London: HMSO.

Michael Report (2008) *Healthcare for All: Independent Inquiry into Access to Healthcare for People with Learning Disabilities.* [online] Available from http://www.iahpld.org.uk/, accessed 12.19.2010.

Mosley J. (1996) *Quality Circle Time in the Primary Classroom: Your Essential Guide to Enhancing Self-esteem, Self-discipline and Positive Relationships.* Cambridge: LDA.

Northern Ireland Executive (2005) *Bamford Review of Mental Health and Learning Disability Equal Lives: Review of Policy and Services for People with a Learning Disability in Northern Ireland.* Belfast: Northern Ireland Executive.

Rogers, C.R. (1957) 'The necessary and sufficient conditions of therapeutic personality change', *Journal of Consulting Psychology*, 21: 95–103.

Scottish Government (2000) *The Same as You? A Review of Services for People with Learning Disabilities.* Edinburgh: The Scottish Government.

Welsh Assembly Government (2007) *Statement on Policy and Practice for Adults with a Learning Disability.* Cardiff: Welsh Assembly Government.

1

SOCIAL POLICY TENSIONS – EMPOWERMENT AND VULNERABILITY

Jonathan Coles

How does recent social policy invite support staff in health and social care settings to understand the implications of having a learning disability?

INTRODUCTION

The twentieth century represented a time of shifting attitudes to disability in general and to people with learning disabilities in particular. This chapter briefly reviews these twentieth century attitude and policy shifts and then looks in more detail at relevant twenty-first century policies which affect the lives of people labelled as having learning disabilities and the practice of those who work with them. New and ostensibly contradictory policies have emerged which simultaneously describe people with learning disabilities as wanting and needing to be empowered, to have more of a say in decision making and in shaping their own lives and services while also being seen as vulnerable to abuse and exploitation and therefore in need of protection. The latter stages will detail examples of good, empowering, safe practice within these policies and will discuss the importance of staff in health and social care settings understanding both the potential vulnerability and the pressing need for empowerment of service users who have learning disabilities.

THE TWENTIETH CENTURY – FROM CONTROL TO CARE

> You weren't allowed out of the hospital. You had to write up and ask could you leave the grounds. You had to ask the medical or write to the doctor and ask them. You couldn't just go across the road and look at the shops; it wasn't allowed unless you wrote up and asked. I didn't go out because I got so used to not going out. You'd get lost if you're not used to it. (Cooper, 1997: 27)

The twentieth century commenced with parliamentary lobbying by powerful eugenicists, demanding that the government tackle the 'problem' of mental deficiency. Eugenicists such as Tredgold believed that many social problems such as prostitution, petty crime and alcoholism were inevitably associated with the 'feeble minded': 'the danger lies in the fact that these degenerates mate with healthy members of the community and thereby constantly drag fresh blood into the vortex of disease and lower the general vigour of the nation.' (Tredgold, 1909: 97).

These negative attitudes to people with learning disabilities, purportedly based in science, were further supported by economics. The Industrial Revolution had brought with it the apparent need to classify people in terms of their ability to contribute to emerging technological and commercial processes and therefore the economic competition between industrialised nations (Race, 1995). People with learning disabilities were considered to be a financial burden because of their lack of skill and intelligence. The Mental Deficiency Act of 1913 gave local authority Mental Deficiency Committees the responsibility to certify and detain the idiots, the imbeciles, the feeble minded and the moral defectives (the newly created official classifications of mental defectives) if care and supervision at home were not thought to be adequate. Over the following twenty years many thousands of people with learning disabilities were compulsorily detained in institutions. These actions were driven by the perceived need to protect society from people with learning disabilities by controlling them (and their ability to procreate). As Goffman (1961) noted, the use of punishment to support conformity was a common feature of institutions.

Wolf Wolfensberger (1972) identified a number of negative socio-historical roles which have been thrust upon people with learning disabilities:

- sub-human organism
- menace
- unspeakable object of dread
- object of pity

- holy innocent
- diseased organism
- object of ridicule
- eternal child.

He states that while these role perceptions reflect prejudice rather than reality, they have nevertheless contributed to the shaping of both our understanding and our social policy in relation to people with learning disabilities.

Reflection Point 1

We have grown up in a society that has negative ideas about people with learning disabilities. How might the terms listed above have influenced how you feel about people with learning disabilities? Do you feel sorry for people, or see them as difficult, or are you inclined to treat them as children? How might your own views of people with learning disabilities influence how you act towards them?

The second half of the twentieth century brought increasingly liberal attitudes towards people with learning disabilities and a shift in the intention and nature of social policy from merely control to concern for their human rights. *The Report of the Royal Commission on the Law Relating to Mental Illness and Mental Deficiency* (Royal Commission, 1957) recommended the expansion of residential, rather than institutional, care and paved the way for the new Mental Health Act (1959), and the discharge of many people with learning disabilities from long-stay institutions – which became hospitals with the advent of the National Health Service – into community settings. The 1960s heralded a number of reports into institutional care in Great Britain which described appalling living conditions and 'custodial attitudes' among staff. The *Report of the Committee of Inquiry into Ely Hospital* (Howe, 1969) was the most significant of these inquiries.

Attitudes towards people with learning disabilities changed rapidly in the final quarter of the twentieth century. With these changes came different social policies and service design principles. In 1971 the White Paper *Better Services for the Mentally Handicapped* (Department of Health and Social Security [DHSS], 1971) recommended a 50 per cent reduction in hospital places by 1991 with increasing local authority residential and day care. It also recommended the re-training of hospital staff. In 1979, The Jay Committee Report advocated the adoption of service philosophies based on the principles of normalisation, defined as the utilisation 'of means which are as culturally normative as possible in order to establish and/or maintain personal behaviours and characteristics which are as culturally normative as possible' (Wolfensberger, 1972: 28).

Normalisation played a significant role in shaping the development of residential and other support services for people with learning disabilities in the UK. In 1991 Wolfensberger renamed and adapted normalisation as 'social role valorisation' (SRV) (Wolfensberger, 1992). SRV had more of a human rights approach and advocated the need to create or support socially valued roles for devalued people on the premise that holding valued social roles leads to the good things which society can offer.

These trends, both in terms of progressive service design principles and community based residential care, were further supported by the National Health Service and Community Care Act (1990).

PROTECTION – A TWENTY-FIRST CENTURY CONCERN

The new millennium brought with it increased governmental concern for the protection of vulnerable adults (including those with learning disabilities). *No Secrets* (DH, 2000) established a national policy for the protection of vulnerable adults. It required local authority social services departments to develop multi-agency codes of practice and offered very clear guidance on the development of local inter-agency policies, procedures and joint protocols. Under this policy, a vulnerable adult is one:

- aged 18 and over
- who may be in need of community care services by reason of mental or other disability, age or illness; and
- who is or may be unable to take care of him or herself, unable to protect him or herself against significant harm or exploitation. (DH, 2000)

Clearly, this policy would cover the majority of people labelled as having learning disabilities, thus establishing both their status as vulnerable and their need for protection from abuse and exploitation. All staff working with people with learning disabilities are required to undergo training in the protection of vulnerable adults which details their responsibility to alert others (social services, health or police) if they have a suspicion or concern that abuse has taken place or might take place if no preventative measures are taken.

In 2005 *No Secrets* and adult protection work in general was further strengthened when the Association of Directors of Social Services (ADSS) published *Safeguarding Adults – A National Framework of Standards for Good Practice and Outcomes in Adult Protection Work* (ADSS, 2005). This sought to collect examples of best practice into a set of practice standards intended as both an audit tool and a guide for adult protection work. Despite this endeavour, investigations into the Cornwall Partnership National Health Service Trust (Healthcare Commission, 2006) and the Sutton and Merton Primary Care Trust (Healthcare Commission, 2007) revealed wide-scale dehumanising treatment of service users with learning disabilities, including incidents of physical and sexual violence and abuse.

While concern for people's safety when they use learning disability services remains high, the increasing number of people with learning disabilities moving into independent living or supported living situations raises additional concerns about bullying and exploitation within the community.

> A hostile reception awaits some, while others are seen as easy pickings for exploitation by people who 'befriend' them and then go on to use their homes, eat their food, steal their money. Although many people need support to live in the community safely and comfortably, there are growing fears that they are not getting it because over-stretched adult services budgets are being used for those with high needs. (Gillen, 2007)

Indeed, the 2006/07 Learning Disabilities Task Force annual report states:

> Evidence shows that people with learning disabilities are often the victims of hate crime. When this happens, they are often not taken seriously by care staff and people working in the Criminal Justice System. This stops people with learning disabilities from reporting hate crime. (Learning Disabilities Task Force, 2007)

These concerns have been validated in the last few years by various incidents of serious bullying against people with learning disabilities which have hit the headlines. In 2009 Fiona Pilkington killed herself and her daughter Francesca, who had learning disabilities, after months of being hounded by local youths. And again:

> In 2007, Christine Lakinski, a woman in her 50s with learning and physical disabilities, was taunted, urinated upon and sprayed with shaving foam as she lay dying in the street. Her brother told me that because of disabilities, she had been picked on for most of her life. (BBC News, 2009)

Also in 2007 a young man with learning disabilities, Brent Martin, was beaten to death by a gang on the estate where he lived in north-east England. The year before this Kevin Davies was imprisoned in a garden shed and tortured horrifically until he died. These horrifying murders are coupled with very high levels of less sensational taunting experienced by people with learning disabilities, 'A *Community Care* survey, published in May, found 16 per cent of almost 2,000 people said they had been bullied on the street in the last year.' (Gillen, 2007). Further research conducted in 2007 involving people with learning disabilities living in supported housing schemes concluded that many tenants had curtailed their participation in social activities because of harassment and they felt unsafe on leaving their homes, especially in the evenings (Fyson et al., 2007). It is quite clear that the need for vigilance and the protection of people with learning disabilities from hate crime and bullying remains.

The new 'personalisation agenda', kick-started by *Putting People First* (Ministers et al., 2007) enables the use of self-directed support and individual budgets, allowing some people with learning disabilities to make better use of existing support networks – friends, family and neighbours – as well as individuals who they recruit and employ to offer particular types of support. Couple this with the steady drift away from residential care into supported living and the picture emerges of a positive new emphasis on personal choice and empowerment. However, Fyson (2009) argues that when increased independence is linked to reduced levels of regulated support, people become more vulnerable because:

- supervision of family, friends and neighbours is problematic
- it can be harder for someone with learning disabilities to complain about family, friends and neighbours
- direct payments and individualised budgets are more open to financial abuse
- protection of vulnerable adults regulations do not apply to those employed via direct payments or individualised budgets
- loneliness can make people vulnerable to being inappropriately befriended.

More recently, *Valuing People Now – A New Three Year Strategy for People with Learning Disabilities* outlines the continuing need to tackle both abuse and hate crime against people with learning disabilities: '...the lives of too many people with learning disabilities are constrained by experience of abuse and neglect and many people have been victims of hate crime.' (DoH, 2009: 108). This re-establishes the need for staff to view people with learning disabilities as vulnerable and accept their own role as protectors.

EMPOWERMENT – THE POLICY BACKGROUND

Self-advocacy groups (of people with learning disabilities) have called for improved services and more involvement and control for people with learning disabilities since People First groups began to form in UK cities. While the precise history of the self-advocacy movement in the UK is difficult to trace,

> UK based self-advocacy is said to have started in 1984 when People First London Boroughs was founded, following the attendance of a small number of people with learning difficulties at the International Conference held in the USA. (Buchanan and Walmesley, 2006: 134)

While local branches of People First determine their own missions and activities, the common agenda is one of empowerment. The information about Bristol and South Gloucestershire People First, available from the South Gloucestershire Council website, starts with the following statement:

> Bristol and South Gloucestershire People First [BSGPF] started as a small group of people with learning difficulties at the Whole Baked Café in Bristol.
>
> We wanted:
>
> - To be in control of our lives
> - Equal rights
> - Proper choices
>
> (BSGPF, no date)

The following is taken from the front page of the national People First website:

> People First promotes the social model of disability. This is a way of thinking about disability that says it is society that needs to change to include disabled people. We should not have to change to fit in with society. We are against the medical model of disability, which is the view that being disabled means there is 'something wrong' with you.
>
> Self-advocacy is people with learning difficulties speaking up for ourselves. Self-advocacy is important because many people with learning difficulties spend their lives being told what to do. If you are always told what to do and never listened to you can get to the point where you don't even know how to make a decision for yourself. (People First, no date)

People First's struggle for more involvement in the shaping of relevant policy was achieved one year after *No Secrets*, when the first White Paper on learning disabilities for thirty years, *Valuing People – A New Strategy for Learning Disabilities for the 21st Century* (DH, 2001) came into force. The White Paper was developed with the involvement of people with learning disabilities and carries a very different message, conveying a progressive view of people with learning disabilities as seeking control over their own lives – empowerment.

There are four 'key principles' at the heart of this policy:

- Legal and Civil Rights: The Government is committed to enforceable civil rights for disabled people in order to eradicate discrimination in society. People with learning disabilities have the right to a decent education, to grow up to vote, to marry and have a family, and to express their opinions, with help and support to do so where necessary ... All public services will treat people with learning disabilities as individuals with respect for their dignity, and challenge discrimination on all grounds including disability. ...
- Independence: Promoting independence is a key aim for the Government's modernisation agenda. ... While people's individual needs will differ, the starting presumption should be one of independence, rather than dependence, with public services providing the support needed to maximise this. Independence in this context does not mean doing everything unaided.
- Choice: Like other people, people with learning disabilities want a real say in where they live, what work they should do and who looks after them. ... This includes people with severe and profound disabilities who, with the right help and support, can make important choices and express preferences about their day to day lives.
- Inclusion: Being part of the mainstream is something most of us take for granted. We go to work, look after our families, visit our GP, use transport, go to the swimming pool or cinema. Inclusion means enabling people with learning disabilities to do those ordinary things ... be fully included in the local community. (DH, 2001: 23–4).

Beyond this the White Paper includes a chapter, 'More Choice and Control for People with Learning Disabilities', which calls for the development of advocacy services including both citizen advocacy and self-advocacy, increased involvement in decision making, improving information and communication with people with learning disabilities and the development of person centred approaches to the planning of services.

A person-centred approach to planning means that planning should start with the individual (not with services), and take account of their wishes and aspirations. Person-centred planning is a mechanism for reflecting the needs and preferences of a person with a learning disability and covers such issues as housing, education, employment and leisure. (DH, 2001: 49)

It also calls for the involvement of service users in both the selection and training of staff who support them.

'I want staff who treat you well, who know how to treat you properly'

The best way to achieve this is to promote the involvement of people with learning disabilities and their family carers in training and development activities. Staff and managers at all levels in organisations need to have an opportunity to hear directly from people with learning disabilities about their expectations. (DH, 2001: 99)

The White Paper also established Learning Disability Partnership Boards in all local authorities with responsibility for overseeing the development of local services for adults with learning disabilities and required to include people with learning disabilities as members.

These principles of choice, involvement and increasing service-user empowerment and control which are advanced within learning disability services by *Valuing People* are also at the heart of recent transformation of adult care policy including *Our Health, Our Care, Our Say* (DH, 2006) and the *Putting People First* agenda (Ministers et al., 2007).

This new social policy concern for the empowerment of people with learning disabilities was given significant support by the Mental Capacity Act (MCA) (2005). The Act sets out fundamental legal rules that apply to everyone working with and/or caring for adults who may lack capacity – including family members, professionals and other carers. The rules also apply to people appointed in a formal capacity to act as an attorney or deputy for a person lacking capacity. It seeks to ensure that all adults are enabled to make any decisions for which they have the capacity to do so. Its underlying philosophy is to ensure that individuals who may lack capacity are the focus of any decisions made, or actions taken, on their behalf. The interests of the person who lacks capacity should prevail, not the views or convenience of those caring for that person.

Reflection Point 2

Do you understand your responsibilities if you believe a person lacks the capacity to make decisions? When you are next at work read your organisational policy on what staff must do if they feel a person lacks capacity to consent.

Many of the provisions in MCA are based upon existing common law principles (i.e. principles that have been established through decisions made by courts in individual cases). MCA 2005 seeks to clarify existing law as well as introduce some new legal safeguards, including new ways in which people can plan ahead for a time when they might lack capacity and the statutory introduction of Independent Mental Capacity Advocates who must be engaged to support people who lack the capacity to make serious decisions about medical treatment or changes of accommodation and who are unbefriended. The Act represents the legal framework and is accompanied by a Code of Practice (Department for Constitutional Affairs [DCA], 2007), which provides guidance and information to those acting under the terms of the legislation. The Code of Practice sets out five statutory principles which are intended to support good practice:

1   A person must be assumed to have capacity unless it is established that they lack capacity.
2   A person is not to be treated as unable to make a decision unless all practicable steps to help him to do so have been taken without success.
3   A person is not to be treated as unable to make a decision merely because he makes an unwise decision.
4   An act done, or decision made, under this Act for or on behalf of a person who lacks capacity must be done, or made, in his best interests.
5   Before the act is done, or the decision is made, regard must be had to whether the purpose for which it is needed can be as effectively achieved in a way that is less restrictive of the person's rights and freedom of action. (DCA, 2007: 19)

The Code of Practice also sets out a simple assessment process which must be employed before anyone concludes that an adult lacks capacity to make a particular decision and subsequently acts in their best interests.

A person is unable to make a decision if they cannot:

1   understand information about the decision to be made (the Act calls this 'relevant information')
2   retain that information in their mind
3   use or weigh that information as part of the decision-making process, or
4   communicate their decision (by talking, using sign language or any other means). (DCA, 2007: 45)

Clearly, decision making lies at the heart of any notions of personal empowerment and if properly enacted this policy brings new power and control to people with learning disabilities. For example, the Code of Practice offers the following scenario to illustrate how someone should be supported as much as possible to make a significant decision for herself:

Scenario

Getting help from other people. Jane has a learning disability. She expresses herself using some words, facial expressions and body language. She has lived in her current community home all her life, but now needs to move to a new group home. She finds it difficult to discuss abstract ideas or things she hasn't experienced. Staff conclude that she lacks the capacity to decide for herself which new group home she should move to. The staff involve an advocate to help Jane express her views. Jane's advocate spends time with her in different environments. The advocate uses pictures, symbols and Makaton to find out the things that are important to Jane, and speaks to people who know Jane to find out what they think she likes. She then supports Jane to show their work to her care manager, and checks that the new homes suggested for her are able to meet Jane's needs and preferences. When the care manager has found some suitable places, Jane's advocate visits the homes with Jane. They take photos of the houses to help her distinguish between them. The advocate then uses the photos to help Jane work out which home she prefers. Jane's own feelings can now play an important part in deciding what is in her best interests – and so in the final decision about where she will live. (DCA, 2007: 38)

And again:

Scenario

Providing relevant information in an appropriate format. Mr Leslie has learning disabilities and has developed an irregular heartbeat. He has been prescribed medication for this, but is anxious about having regular blood tests to check his medication levels. His doctor gives him a leaflet to explain:

the reason for the tests,
what a blood test involves,
the risks in having or not having the tests, and
that he has the right to decide whether or not to have the test.

The leaflet uses simple language and photographs to explain these things. Mr Leslie's carer helps him read the leaflet over the next few days and checks that he understands it. Mr Leslie goes back to tell the doctor that, even though he is scared of needles, he will agree to the blood tests so that he can get the right medication. He is able to pick out the equipment needed to do the blood test. So the doctor concludes that Mr Leslie can understand, retain and use the relevant information and therefore has the capacity to make the decision to have the test. (DCA, 2007: 47)

Despite this focus on decision making and support for empowerment, the MCA also concerns itself with the issue of protection and the Code of Practice includes a chapter, 'What means of protection exist for people who lack capacity to make decisions for themselves?' This describes the different agencies that exist to ensure that adults who lack capacity to make decisions for themselves are protected from abuse and sets out what somebody should do if they suspect that somebody is abusing a vulnerable adult who lacks capacity. It also introduces two new criminal offences: ill treatment and wilful neglect of a person who lacks capacity to make relevant decisions. It offers the following scenario to illustrate who should become involved in ascertaining whether someone with a learning disability is making a capacitated decision, or else perhaps being exploited, assaulted or abused:

Scenario

Involving professional opinion. Ms Ledger is a young woman with learning disabilities and some autistic spectrum disorders. Recently she began a sexual relationship with a much older man, who is trying to persuade her to move in with him and come off the pill. There are rumours that he has been violent towards her and has taken her bankbook. Ms Ledger boasts about the relationship to her friends. But she has admitted to her key worker that she is sometimes afraid of the man. Staff at her sheltered accommodation decide to make a referral under the local adult protection procedures. They arrange for a clinical psychologist to assess Ms Ledger's understanding of the relationship and her capacity to consent to it. (DCA, 2007: 60)

Clearly, staff could have responded differently here. If they had prioritised Ms Ledger's autonomy and empowerment this could have obscured the possibility that she is being abused. What matters here is the question of her capacity to consent to sexual activity. If this is established, she has the legal right to determine this for herself; if not, she has the right to protection.

Reflection Point 3

You are a practice nurse and are doing an annual health check and health action plan for an individual with learning disabilities.

Paul is a 52 year old man who has Down's syndrome and has lived in this home for 12 years after spending most of his early life in a long-stay institution. One of Paul's favourite activities is going to the pub, which he does three times each week (with support to get there and back, but no support while he is there), usually drinking 3 or 4 pints of strong beer. While Paul has no contact with family, 3 years ago he was left a substantial amount of money by an auntie. He manages a weekly budget of 'spending money' by himself – £95, covering outings, holidays, magazines, beer, clothes etc.

Paul communicates effectively with people who know him well using some spoken language, photographs (arranged into sections in a folder – food, people, activities, feelings, etc).

Recently staff at the home have been concerned about Paul. His short-term memory seems to be weakening and his concentration span reducing. He is less communicative generally and occasionally acts out of character. You arrange a visit to the GP which has resulted in tests indicating that Paul is in the early stages of vascular dementia – possibly connected, in part, with alcohol consumption. The GP has strongly recommended that Paul should give up alcohol. Paul is keen to continue his trips to the pub and his consumption of beer.

What are your concerns at this stage?

How might you help the home to establish whether Paul has the capacity to make this decision for himself?

If he does not have capacity to make this decision for himself, how would you try to establish Paul's best interests?

CONCLUSION

Modern social policy offers two lenses through which staff in health and social care settings might view people with learning disabilities. One lens prioritises empowerment, autonomy and self-determination; the other highlights the potential vulnerability of adults with learning disabilities to abuse – within specialist services and in society in general. Sensitive, empowering practice requires staff to hold both of these perspectives in focus, without prioritising one over the other. A lack of sensitivity and vigilance can allow exploitation, neglect and abuse to become part of the everyday, taken-for-granted life experience of people with learning disabilities. As with risk aversive risk management practice, an over-protective attitude will disempower and diminish people's lives. Service providers need to have a clear understanding of individual rights, rigorous capacity assessment, opportunities for both staff and service users to learn and develop, and staff who understand their roles as supporting people with learning disabilities to take control of their own lives wherever possible, while staying alert to the reality of vulnerability.

Social care can and should be provided in such a way as to enable adults with learning disabilities to be as independent as they are able, and to have real choices in their lives. However, independence should not be promoted dogmatically. There must also be a recognition that people who receive adult social care services because they have a learning disability are more vulnerable to abuse than other citizens. (Fyson, 2009: 23)

Changing patterns of adult social care, and particularly the increasing numbers of people with learning disabilities who live with greater freedoms and independence and less support from paid staff, place an even greater significance on getting this balance right.

⚷ Key Learning Points ⚷

- During the twentieth century many people with learning disabilities experienced oppression
- Towards the end of the twentieth century things began to improve with the move from institutional care to residential care and 'ordinary living' principles
- The twenty-first century commenced with increasing governmental concern for the involvement and empowerment of people with learning disabilities
- Recent policies and research highlight the need for the protection of people with learning disabilities from crime, abuse and exploitation as their freedoms and community presence increase.

REFERENCES

Association of Directors of Social Services (ADSS) (2005) *Safeguarding Adults – A National Framework of Standards for Good Practice and Outcomes in Adult Protection Work*. London: The Association of Directors of Social Services.

BBC News (2009) 'Spotlight on disability hate crime', 29 September 2009. [website] Available from http://news.bbc.co.uk/1/hi/uk/8280577.stm.

Bristol and South Gloucestershire People First (no date) *Bristol and South Gloucestershire People First*. [online] Available from http://www.southglos.gov.uk/NR/exeres/9b17742c-c7d5-493c-aca2-5498121d09c5, accessed 27.3.2010.

Buchanan, I. and Walmsley, J. (2006) 'Self-advocacy in historical perspective', *British Journal of Learning Disabilities*, 34: 133–8.

Cooper, M. (1997) 'Forgotten lives', in: D. Atkinson, M. Jackson and J. Walmsley (eds), *Forgotten Lives: Exploring the History of Learning Disability*. Kidderminster: British Institute of Learning Disabilities.

Department for Constitutional Affairs (2007) *Mental Capacity Act 2005 Code of Practice*. London: Department for Constitutional Affairs.

Department of Health (2000) *No Secrets: Guidance on Developing and Implementing Multi-agency Policies and Procedures to Protect Vulnerable Adults from Abuse.* London: Department of Health.

Department of Health (2001) *Valuing People: A New Strategy for Learning Disability for the 21st Century.* London: Department of Health.

Department of Health (2006) *Our Health, Our Care, Our Say.* London: Department of Health.

Department of Health (2009) *Valuing People Now – A New Three Year Strategy for People with Learning Disabilities.* London: Department of Health.

Department of Health and Social Security (1971) *Better Services for the Mentally Handicapped.* Cm. 4683. London: HMSO.

Fyson, R. (2009) 'Independence and learning disabilities: why we must also recognise vulnerability', *The Journal of Adult Protection,* 11 (3): 18–25.

Fyson, R., Tarleton, B. and Ward, L. (2007) *Support for Living? The Impact of the Supporting People Programme on Housing and Support for Adults with Learning Disabilities.* Bristol/York: Policy Press/Joseph Rowntree Foundation.

Gillen, S. (2007) 'How People with Learning Disabilities Face Bullying and Harassment' Thursday 27 September *Community Care.* [online] Available from http://www.communitycare.co.uk/Articles/2007/09/27/105921/how-people-with-learning-disabilities-face-bullying-and-harassment.htm, accessed 17.03.2011.

Goffman, E. (1961) *Asylums: Essays on the Social Situation of Mental Patients and other Inmates.* Harmondsworth: Penguin.

Jay Committee (1979) *Report of the Committee of Enquiry into Mental Handicap Nursing and Care.* Cm. 7468. London: HMSO.

Healthcare Commission (2006) *Joint Investigation into the Provision of Services for People with Learning Disabilities at Cornwall Partnership NHS Trust.* London: Healthcare Commission.

Healthcare Commission (2007) *Investigation into the Service for People with Learning Disabilities Provided by Sutton and Merton Primary Care Trust.* London: Healthcare Commission.

Howe, G. (1969) *'Report of the Committee of Inquiry into Ely Hospital'* (Howe Report). [online] Available from http://www.sochealth.co.uk/history/Ely.htm, accessed 30.06.2010.

Learning Disabilities Task Force (2007) Annual Report 2006–7. [online] Available from http://www.dh.gov.uk/prod_consum_dh/groups/dh_digitalassets/@dh/@en/documents/digitalasset/dh_078362.pdf, accessed 17.03.2011.

Mental Capacity Act (2005) London: HMSO.

Mental Deficiency Act (1913) London: HMSO.

Mental Health Act (1959) London: HMSO.

Ministers, local government, NHS, social care, professional and regulatory organisations (2007) *Putting People First: A Shared Vision and Commitment to the Transformation of Adult Social Care.* London: Department of Health.

National Health Service and Community Care Act (1990) London: HMSO.

People First (no date) *What is People First?* [online] Available from http://www.people-firstltd.com. accessed 27.03.2010.

Race, D. (1995) 'Historical development of service provision', in N. Malin (ed.), *Services for People with Learning Disabilities*. London: Routledge.

Royal Commission (1957) *Report of the Royal Commission on the Law Relating to Mental Illness and Mental Deficiency: 1954–57*. Cm.169. London: HMSO.

Tredgold, A.F. (1909) 'The feebleminded – a social danger' *Eugenics Review*, 1: 97–104.

Wolfensberger, W. (1972) *The Principle of Normalization in Human Services*. Toronto: National Institute on Mental Retardation.

Wolfensberger, W. (1992) *A Brief Introduction to Social Role Valorization as a High-order Concept for Structuring Human Services*. Syracuse, New York: Training Institute for Human Service Planning, Leadership and Change Agency.

2

THE HISTORY AND CONTEXT OF LEARNING DISABILITY: A PARENT'S PERSPECTIVE

Jackie Edwards

INTRODUCTION

This chapter explores a parent's perspective of the cultural changes in the way people with a learning disability are supported and how services have developed over the past forty years. A cultural change of accepting and including everyone as they are, rather than attempting to cure or change the individual, has meant that the medical model of care and large hospitals have been replaced with a social model of care in the community. Parliamentary reform bills, informed by self-advocates and families, have reinforced the rights of individuals to have greater choice and control over how they are supported. Changes in language and terminology have also contributed to a change in perception, for example the term 'mentally handicapped' has been replaced with 'learning disability' or 'learning difficulty'. All these changes are moving professions from seeing an individual as needing to be cared for to seeing a person as needing to be supported so that they can be as independent as they are able to be and free to develop their own interests through the personalisation agenda.

The chapter will offer a brief history of learning disability legislation over the last forty years, provide a discussion of the medical and social models of disability from a parent's perspective, and explore the moves toward inclusion and inclusive practice. It will discuss person centred planning and the personalisation agenda, in addition to some perceived pressures that exist between professionals and families. This chapter provides some valuable insights into how families are struggling with rapidly changing philosophies and how a locus of control is shifting from professionals to families to meet the needs of their family member.

A BRIEF HISTORY OF LEARNING DISABILITY POLICY

A number of reports and legislative Acts have informed and driven the direction of change over the last four decades. *Better Services for the Mentally Handicapped* (Department of Health and Social Security, 1971) was instrumental in starting the move from institutional care to community care. Philosophical change through the introduction of normalisation theory and Social Role Valorisation (SRV) during the 1970s and 1980s (Wolfensberger 1972, 1998, 2007) contributed to a major service change introduced through the National Health Service and Community Care Act (1990). This focussed on improved support within the community rather than the traditional support provided by the learning disability institutions across the UK. Eleven years later this was followed by the White Paper, *Valuing People: A New Strategy for Learning Disability for the 21st Century* (Department of Health (DH) 2001). *Valuing People* set out how the government intended to provide new opportunities for children and adults with learning disabilities and their families to live full and independent lives as part of their local communities. This agenda was strengthened by the personalisation agenda in the government papers *Our Health, Our Care, Our Say* (DH, 2006), and *Putting People First* (Ministers et al., 2007). These papers set out to give people with a learning disability and their family carers the chance to have a real say in the planning, purchasing and monitoring of services. Many of the changes in policy and practice have been in response to the increased impact of the Human Rights Act (1998) and the European Convention of Human Rights and Fundamental Freedoms (Council of Europe, 2010). These emphasised the need to address the range of inequalities experienced by people with a learning disability and their families. They also clarified that services and agencies have a responsibility to take appropriate action as and when necessary to maintain people's rights. Families have looked on from the sidelines trying to keep up with the pace of change, often becoming confused by the implications and impact of legislation on the services and supports that they and their family member can expect.

CONTEMPORARY POLICY

Death by Indifference, a Mencap report (2007), told the stories of six people with learning disabilities whom Mencap believed died unnecessarily due to discrimination in the NHS. This report led to the *Independent Inquiry into Access to Healthcare for People with Learning Disabilities* (Michael Report, 2008). These reports highlighted how the NHS failed to uphold people's rights and needed to change in order that the needs of people with learning disabilities could be met. Concurrently the Joint Committee on Human Rights report, *A Life Like Any Other?*, stated that:

> The Committee expects the Government to give the recommendations in this Report serious consideration when it redrafts the current consultation document *Valuing People Now*. It recommends that *Valuing People Now* should promote a human rights based approach and provide practical guidance to public authorities on how human rights principles can be used to secure better treatment. (2008: 5)

Valuing People Now (DH, 2009) retained the original vision of *Valuing People* (DH, 2001) but set it firmly within the context of a number of significant recent reports published in the first decade of the twenty-first century, including:

- *Death by Indifference* (Mencap, 2007)
- *Aiming High for Disabled Children and their Families* (DfES, 2007)
- *Healthcare for All* (Michael Report, 2008)
- *Putting People First* report (Ministers et al., 2007)
- *Carers at the Heart of Twenty-first Century Families and Communities* (DH, 2008)
- *A Life Like Any Other?* (Joint Committee on Human Rights, 2008)

As such, *Valuing People Now* (DH, 2009) emphasises a key element of delivery to be the development of capacity and capability at local levels to design and commission services that people need. These services should enable people to live healthy, independent lives, close to their families and friends. Local partnership with people with learning disabilities and their families is stressed as crucial, as is the formation of Learning Disability Partnership Boards (LDPB), highlighting their vital role in service development. For example, family carer and self-advocate representatives sit on their local LDPB and the various sub-groups considering access to health services, housing options, opportunities for employment and personalisation. The representatives sitting on the LDPB are invited to confirm the annual self-assessment reports, thus offering them an opportunity to participate in local plans and decision making.

Family carers and self-advocates are also able to feed back through the regional and national forums directly to government ministers.

Reflection Point 4

Think about the Mencap statement that staff in the NHS discriminate against people with learning disabilities.

What behaviours and actions do you think show that someone is discriminating against another person? You might want to consider the language people use, the 'jokes' they tell, as well as withholding or delaying treatment.

Think about yourself; do you believe people with learning disabilities have equal rights to access healthcare?

If you do believe in equal rights, how might you challenge someone who is being discriminatory?

If you believe people with learning difficulties do not have the same rights, be honest with yourself and consider how you will guard against your personal beliefs leading to poor healthcare for a person you are caring for.

THE MEDICAL AND SOCIAL MODELS OF DISABILITY

An integral part of this growing focus on human rights has been the use of language and terminology highlighting the need to ensure that a person is not defined in terms of their disability. An awareness of each person as a whole is now required, acknowledging their strengths and needs, rather than attempting to fit them into rigid diagnostic criteria. In the UK this history of rapidly changing terminology has often caused some difficulty for families in keeping up with what's current and 'in vogue'. The use of terminology across different agencies and professional groups remains variable. For example, there has been an ongoing debate about the use of the terms learning difficulty and learning disability. Significantly, how terminology is used and interpreted can make a difference as to whether a person is included or excluded from service provision. For example, 'learning difficulty' tends to suggest service eligibility for individuals with neurological differences such as Asperger's Syndrome, Dyslexia, and Attention Deficit Hyperactivity Disorder (ADHD), while 'learning disability' is the language used in health service provision.

The context of change is more than simply the language and descriptors used. The medical model of disability provides the traditional model upon which many of our established values, attitudes, practices and service structures are founded. The premise that the person has an illness or disability that can be cured or that results in the need for care provision gives rise to the belief that any such disability has a negative effect on an individual's quality of life. As a result, curing or managing illness or disability involves identifying the illness or disability, understanding it and learning to control and alter its course (Open University, 2006a). To promote a more normal life the medical model advocates that we change the individual to fit into society to promote a 'normal' life. Thus, as a just society – within the context of this model – we are driven to invest resources in healthcare and related services in an attempt to 'cure' disabilities medically.

In 'Internalised Oppression' Mason describes the impact of the medical model from the perspective of a disabled person. She writes:

> You have just struggled out into the world fully expecting a warm welcome, but instead you get 'Oh God! How could this happen to me? Aaargh!' How do you think this would make you feel about yourself? Good? No, of course not. The medical model of disability leads from the point of diagnosis to a lifetime of feeling that we are a disappointment and a worry to everyone. It seems perfectly logical to conclude that having a disability is a bad thing because it upsets everyone, and eliminating or lessening the disability is a worthwhile obsession because without it, you as a person will be a joy to those you love most, instead of misery. (Mason, 1990: 2)

Within the context of the medical model, disabled people and their medical practitioners are often left feeling like failures. A continual cycle of failing to be cured can lead to loss of self-esteem, confidence, motivation in the disabled person, and frustration for the professionals. Of even deeper concern is the total impact the disability, when viewed from this perspective, has on a person's life. Mason (1990) goes on to say: 'Other children play, but you do "therapy". Other children develop, but you are "trained". Almost every activity of daily living can take on the dimension of trying to make you less like yourself and more like the able-bodied' (1990: 2).

The dominance of the medical model in relation to the support of disabled people remained unchallenged until the 1960s and even then the impact of the social model upon the lives of people with a learning disability was negligible. The UK organisation Union of the Physically Impaired Against Segregation (UPIAS) claimed that disability was: 'the disadvantage or restriction of activity caused by a contemporary social organisation which takes little or no account of people who have physical impairments and thus excludes them from participation in the mainstream of social activities' (UPIAS, 1976: 3). This was the point at which the term 'social model of disability' was coined and was largely as a result of the work of disabled academic Mike Oliver (1987, 1990). Rather than focussing on treatment and cure, the social model of disability requires society to readjust in relation to the barriers that prevent the inclusion and participation of disabled people. The social model of disability proposes that it is the systemic barriers, negative attitudes and exclusion by society – purposely or inadvertently – that define who is disabled and who is not. The social model acknowledges that people may have physical, sensory, intellectual, or psychological differences that can cause individual functional limitation. However, the model suggests that these do not have to lead to disability; rather, if society takes account of the access needs of all it's citizens and adapts to include people regardless of such individual differences people are not disabled (Open University, 2006b).

The social model of disability implies that attempts to 'change', 'fix' or 'cure' individuals, especially when against the wishes of the person, can be discriminatory and prejudiced. Furthermore, to disadvantage a person's access or inclusion, either actively or by the absence of provision, became legally challengeable through the Disability Discrimination Act (1995, 2005). Upon its introduction, the Act aimed to end the discrimination that many disabled people faced. The Act has since been succeeded by the Equalities Act (2010).

An example of the move from the medical to social model can be seen in the use of medication to manage challenging behaviour for those with a severe learning disability. The desire to control and change the individual by using drugs is slowly being replaced by functional assessments that consider environmental factors and seek to provide appropriate support to enable inclusion (Challenging Behaviour Foundation, 2010).

The continuing push to adopt the social model is influencing the range of services and support approaches offered to people with learning disabilities and their families. The advent of the social model has also prompted a greater emphasis on ability and capacity, moving away from the former focus on deficit and problem. However, papers such as *Valuing People Now* (DH, 2009) indicate that society has been slow to adjust and many preconceived ideas and judgements remain, despite the attention given to the issues.

Significantly, changes from the medical to social model focussed on making tangible changes to the messages that parents receive upon recognition that their child has a disability. For example, the language used has generally moved away from encouraging acceptance of the 'tragic' situation toward more hopefulness and positive expectations for the child's future (see Chapter 5). Then, as the child becomes recognised as a child with complex and additional needs, so services are developed to assist inclusion within the context of the family, the local community and locally provided specialist supports (see Chapter 4).

Reflection Point 5

Consider the last time you supported an individual with any form of disability. Which model was emphasised more in the caring of that person?

Where do you consider your own practice to be in relation to these two models?

MOVING TOWARDS INCLUSION

Education

The progression of inclusive education has led to educational services adopting a prominent role during the school age years. There has been a move away from the segregated education of disabled children described by Warnock (1978) through to their inclusion in mainstream provision (Education Act 1981, 1993). The Special Educational Needs and Disability Act (2001) made it unlawful for schools in the UK to discriminate against children with disabilities and obliged local education authorities to assess children's needs to ensure they received individual support to access education. This was followed by the Education (Disability Strategies and Pupils' Educational Records) (Scotland) Act (2002), requiring Scottish schools to have accessibility plans in place. Children's rights to inclusive education have now been enshrined in the UN Convention on the Rights of Persons with Disabilities (UN, 2006). It has been thought that making the change in children's services will have the best possibility of influencing the desired cultural change. However, while some local authorities have chosen to adopt total mainstream education policies, closing all their special schools and investing heavily in inclusion, others have assured the principle that parents should retain the right to exercise choice through the retention of segregated education (Abbott, Morris and Ward, 2001). Therefore, the impact of policy change has varied geographically, but equally there is a wide variety of parental aspirations.

Using Community Facilities

There has been a growing awareness of the need for social and extracurricular support to enable people with learning disabilities to access their communities. Indeed one of the *Valuing People* (DH, 2001) goals was to modernise day services and increase community involvement. The success of such ventures depends on the provision of appropriate supports that enable individuals and their families to participate (e.g. personal assistants, buddy schemes). For the disabled person it is important that choices include the range of local, community-based activities and opportunities and can select activities in just the same way as any other citizen would. It is also important that the groups they wish to join are able and willing to make it a positive experience. However, the Learning Disability Coalition (2007) highlights that the reality is that, despite day service closures, people are not always supported to access their communities but have to stay at home.

Health

People with learning disabilities have the same rights to good healthcare as any member of society. In response to *Death by Indifference* (Mencap, 2007) and *Healthcare for All* (Michael Report, 2008) the role of the hospital liaison nurse has developed. These nurses usually have a qualification in nursing people with learning disabilities and have a remit to improve both access to healthcare and the patient's experience of receiving healthcare and to promote effective discharge. A significant role is the education of healthcare staff to improve their knowledge of how to support people with learning disabilities (Buchanan, 2011).

Removing barriers

With barriers to inclusion preventing people living their lives, there is a need to support communities to be inclusive. This would suggest that the work of community-based learning disability services is to support the range of social, leisure and learning opportunities through the provision of information, training and direct action. There is some evidence that this is indeed happening. For example, some local authorities and health and social care providers are enabling their staff to undertake specifically designed training. (e.g. Social Inclusion Training available from the National Development Team for Inclusion: http://www.ndti.org.uk).
Also, one council has employed people with learning disabilities as inclusion champions to provide training to organisations within their communities (South Gloucestershire Council, 2010).

A PARENT PERSPECTIVE OF PERSON CENTRED PLANNING

Much of the change witnessed for people with learning disabilities and their families since the 1980s has been underpinned by the introduction of person centred approaches and person centred planning. Inclusive Solutions, an organisation developed out of the work of Colin Newton and Derek Wilson in relation to inclusive practice in one local authority, offers the following description:

> Person Centred Planning is built on the values of inclusion and looks at what support a person needs to be included and involved in their community. Person centred approaches offer an alternative to traditional types of planning which are based upon the medical model of disability and which are set up to assess need, allocate services and make decisions for people. Person centred planning is rooted in the social model and aims to empower people who have traditionally been disempowered by 'specialist' or segregated services by handing power and control back to them. (Inclusive Solutions, no date)

During the 1990s there were numerous examples of people and their families, not-for-profit organisations, groups and individuals actively promoting the need to deliver on person centred approaches and planning. *Valuing People* (DH, 2001) firmly rooted its importance within the context of services offered to people with a learning disability. Just as progress by services regarding person centred planning has varied, so has the progress and impact experienced by people and their families (Robertson et al., 2007).

The community organisation Circles Network, founded in 1994, addressed family and community work with effective use of person centred planning. First developed in Canada, circles of support were brought to the UK by Circles Network (http://www.circlesnetwork.org.uk) in partnership with the organisation Communitas almost twenty years ago. The idea of a 'circle' is that effort is invested in building up a group of committed people around an isolated individual (and their family if relevant). The group offer non-judgemental support to the person, supplying human friendship, companionship and support. They become allies in the push for rightful inclusion and empowerment. Person centred planning is used as a fundamental tool in helping the person identify aspirations and plan the steps towards achieving them.

Reaching out to people and their families in this way, Circles Network paved the way for a series of further initiatives based on the concept that people themselves are in the best position to be describing the supports that would make best sense to them. This is in direct contrast to the more traditional model of fitting people into a defined service which inevitably ends up organised around the needs of the organisation and those working for it. Additionally, people in the person's life who love them, know them well and understand their subtle communications can be strong allies in enabling the person to achieve their goals.

However, when the role of person centred planning facilitator has been placed with support staff, there is anecdotal evidence from families feeding back through family carer forum meetings that some organisations struggle to engage with them, and that they feel that they are being marginalised and excluded from the process. There is a sense that some organisations, services and families are challenged by the concept of change – for example, that a person has the right to make a mistake or choose something that they may not necessarily agree with. This includes forming relationships and allowing the individual to take a risk and maybe experience a rejection as part of their journey towards discovering who they are and what their values and goals in life would be.

The premise of using person centred planning to support the development of a support plan and a personalised budget is intended to simplify the process and enable people to make more relevant decisions as to how money can be best used to support them to achieve a good life, on their terms. However, a number of pressing issues hinders the progress of personalisation (DH, 2009).

During the early part of the twenty-first century the concept known as 'personalisation' (giving choice and control to the individual) was taken forward by people active in the field of learning disability and who were supported by the values and initiatives introduced through *Valuing People* (DH, 2001). People seeking to improve the lives of disabled people and their families founded the registered charity In Control in 2003 (In Control, 2011). It was established to find a new way of organising the social care system, with a particular focus on the self-directed support model being developed in collaboration with disabled people, families and social care professionals. For many people being in the driving seat of how their personal support is organised and delivered is not a new idea. However, for other families this has created anxiety as they struggle to keep up with the ideology and question why there needs to be change, especially older family carers who have spent many years adjusting to the traditional approaches.

For the professionals who are tasked with managing this cultural change the experience of the introduction of the In Control model has been dependent on the resources, understanding and policy of the local authority in which they work. In Control's support and advice to the government led to the *Putting People First* policy (Ministers et al., 2007), which set out to transform adult social care. The aim of *Putting People First* is to change the way social care services are provided so that people who use services and carers have greater control and choice about the services they receive.

FAMILIES LIVING WITH CHANGE

There have been many changes for people with a learning disability and their families to adjust to as the political expectation driven by active campaigners for community support has continued to advocate for people's right to live ordinary lives as citizens in their community. Certainly, there is a much greater emphasis on the expert role of parents and family members as main carers, which is welcomed by some families but for others remains an area of anxiety, especially in relation to changing service (Cox, 2008). Anecdotal feedback from family carer support groups suggests that families and the individual with a learning disability may not always agree (Partners in Policymaking (PiP), 2010). For example, how independent an individual would like to be may depend on how well their families are able to adjust to the new culture of supporting them in the community. This poignantly raises the issue of the level of vulnerability of those people in our society who are not afforded access to advocacy support. Conversely, families usually make good advocates and when the same degree of advocacy and support as provided by families does not exist, the person with a learning disability may have no-one in their life to be there for them in this way and support them to live the life they want (Robertson et al., 2007). This is particularly important for those who are described as having challenging behaviour (Challenging Behaviour Foundation, 2010). With the best of intentions, support staff often believe they can serve the function of friend, family and advocate. However, this rarely actually happens as staff have dual loyalties and are restrained by professional boundaries that make it difficult for them to offer a lifelong commitment, where a real and lasting relationship has been allowed to flourish and grow. Therefore, staff move in and out of people's lives without establishing any of the ties and long-term connections that exist in a mutual and respectful two-way relationship.

The amount and degree of change in philosophy and service delivery has had varied impact, dependent upon the situation for each individual and their family. Families have expressed their concerns about the changes, especially some older carers who have supported their family member for many years and who are struggling to come to terms with recent changes due to the day service modernisation agenda (Cox, 2008). From my experience of talking with carers, the perceived U-turn in service philosophy leaves them bewildered as to whether they 'did something wrong' for all the years they used segregated, excluding services (e.g. day centres, respite care units and Gateway clubs). They are confused by the message that meaningful days include supporting people into paid employment, when in their lifetime their family member was considered uneducable, never mind employable. They watch young people today now going to college and being supported towards employment with a sense of knowing that their family member could have achieved more but are now past being able to benefit from the new culture and improved opportunities available. The changes made in provision may have resulted in their family member being home more than they were before. Family carers may find that they are now back to cooking a main meal that previously their family member would have received at the day centre. Other family carers are reporting that they are finding it difficult to help their son or daughter to get sufficient exercise now as some local authorities have become focussed on employment and learning activities.

For younger carers of people with a learning disability there are different confusions. They have grown with the inclusion agenda only to discover that the world of services and supports may not yet be ready or able to deliver this safely and successfully for all disabled children and adults in our society. The personalisation agenda suggests that they and their family member can have the choice and control previously the domain of the professional expert. Some stories illustrate great success where this is achieved in a cooperative partnership arrangement (Clarke et al., 2007). Families look to those stories of success and see 'it can be done'. Yet the truth is that for many of the successes achieved the degree of strength, knowledge and determination by the person, their family (and often the circle of support) has been the key factor in determining the positive out-come. For many more families the experience proves to be frustrating and unwieldy as they negotiate their way through the various manifestations of the implementation of In Control (www.in-control.org.uk) and *Putting People First* (Ministers et al., 2007) within their own local authority.

From a family point of view it can be perceived that the new structures and processes are only possible if they take on yet more in the way of support – often in ways that are unfamiliar and uncomfortable. For example, *Putting People First* (Ministers et al., 2007) emphasises better utilisation of friend-ships, relationships and communities in supporting people to achieve inclusive and preferred lifestyles. However, in the absence of any concerted or coordinated effort to invest in and develop communities towards this aim, it is left to families to see this as meaning they will need to provide care and support when services 'don't, won't or can't'. With focus on self-directed support, families may feel that the obligation will be on them to help their family member 'be in control' of their supports and how they are arranged. Managing money and employment matters is dependent on an individual's capacity and level of support needs. It is not the suggestion of *Putting People First* (Ministers et al., 2007) that any person should feel obligated or under pressure to do these things. However, the difficulty most often experienced is that the services people and their families/carers turn to and wish to rely upon, are not yet able to deliver the agenda in an effective manner. Professionals were previously the decision makers and therefore in control. The person and their families/carers were passive recipients of services. This represents a power shift that some professionals and service providers as well as families are finding difficult.

Reflection Point 6

Think about how your life would change if you needed to take on the care of an adult in your family.

Would you feel skilled in managing their health and social care budgets, employing staff (don't forget payroll and the CRB checks) while also providing ongoing support for them to access the community and stay healthy and safe?

What would you want provided to help you do these tasks?

FAMILIES AS LEADERS

With the shift in power discussed above, it has been recognised that families and people with learning disabilities need access to training to take on their newly developing role. The number of leadership courses for parents and disabled adults has grown in the UK, the most notable of these courses are provided by Partners in Policymaking (PiP, 2010). PiP originated in the USA as a result of the work of Colleen Wieck who recognised that it tended to be the parents of disabled children and adults who went to meetings and formed groups. They did not appear to work with the self-advocacy movement or with people who work for services. She also saw that parents and self-advocates did not always agree with each other and that this often meant that the people making the decisions heard different messages from different groups. This lack of consensus made it difficult to progress change in the services offered. PiP was designed as a way of ensuring that the groups could communicate and work together, preparing the right information in order to negotiate their way through meetings successfully (PiP, 2010).

Since the introduction of Partners in Policymaking in the UK, the organisation – led by Lyn Elwell – has grown and has expanded the range of leadership training opportunities it now offers. Courses include:

- Sharing the Challenges – Embracing the needs of parents of people 16 years of age and above
- Tomorrow's Leaders – supporting self-advocates
- Sharing Knowledge – Parents of children 14–19 years of age can plan with their child for their future as an adult
- Kindred Spirits – Providing a course for a range of people working in services and parents who share the goal of working towards desirable futures for disabled children.

CONCLUSION

Over the course of the past forty years the changes in the approaches to working with people with learning disabilities, from the use of language and terminology to the perceptions of how people want to be supported, have developed and been informed by self-advocates and families. A cultural change of accepting and including everyone as they are rather than attempting to cure or change an individual so that they can fit into society has meant that the large hospitals and the medical model of care have been replaced with a social model of care in the community. Parliamentary reform bills have reinforced the rights of individuals to have a greater degree of choice and control over their support. The cultural changes have developed at different levels depending on the services and families involved. For example, children's services have been able to make adjustments to education that may have raised aspirations for younger families, whereas older families may have found it more difficult to understand the changes or may be less able to adapt to new ways of working, such as their son or daughter living in the community.

Service providers have also had to adapt how they provide services. For example a focus on personalisation will have a financial impact on how they manage funding and staffing so that individuals can choose, rather than fit into organised service-led activities and opportunities. They have had to develop partnerships, working closely with families and the local authority to ensure that they are adjusting to a new way of working. Local authorities have set up Learning Disability Partnership Boards that include family carers and self-advocates as well as other stakeholders to ensure that their voices are heard when developing services. However, not all families are able to access forum meetings or are able to give a voice to their concerns for a variety of reasons. Therefore, representation remains limited to those who are able to participate.

The move towards inclusion remains a cultural change in the process of being developed rather than a completed achievement. *Valuing People Now* (DH, 2009) suggests that by 2011 many of the basic principles, such as living where a person chooses and with whom, having access to equality within the health services, and employment opportunities when possible, should be available. For some individuals with a learning disability this remains an aspiration rather than an achievable outcome. How services develop to meet the challenge of a person centred service will be an evolving process.

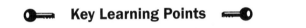

Key Learning Points

- The rapidly changing policy context, while necessary for inclusion, can be daunting for those people who are directly affected by such rapid change
- Cultural changes in perception from a medical to a social model of disability are helping people to change their views on what disability means
- Inclusive communities are starting to develop but this will take time
- Being person centred is central to people being enabled to live their own life
- Listening and learning are important when working with people with learning disabilities and their families.

REFERENCES

Abbott. D., Morris. J. and Ward, L. (2001) *The Best Place to Be? Policy, Practice and the Experiences of Residential School Placements for Disabled Children.* Bristol: The Norah Fry Research Centre.

Buchanan, D. (2011) 'Learning disabilities awareness training for hospital staff', *Nursing Times* (in press).

Challenging Behaviour Foundation (2010) *A Guide for Advocates: Supporting People with Learning Disabilities who are Described as Having Challenging Behaviour.* Kent: The Challenging Behaviour Foundation.

Clarke, J., Seamer, J., Jones, D. and Scarborough, K. (2007) 'Trusting people: families leading services', *PMLD Link*, 19 (1): 7–10.

Council of Europe (2010) 'Convention for the Protection of Human Rights and Fundamental Freedoms as amended by Protocols No. 11 and No. 14' (original

1950, updated 2010). [online] Available from http://conventions.coe.int/Treaty/EN/Treaties/html/005.htm, accessed 30.06.2010.

Cox, J. (2008) *Response To Valuing People Now Consultation*. Bristol: National Family Carer Network.

Department for Education and Skills (2007) *Aiming High for Disabled Children: Better Support for Families*. London: Department for Education and Skills.

Department of Health (2001) *Valuing People: A New Strategy for Learning Disability for the 21st Century*. London: Department of Health.

Department of Health (2006) *Our health, our care, our say: a new direction for community services*. London: Department of Health.

Department of Health (2008) *Carers at the Heart of 21st-century Families and Communities*. London: Department of Health.

Department of Health (2009) *Valuing People Now: A New Three Year Strategy for People with Learning Disabilities*. London: Department of Health.

Department of Health and Social Security (1971) *Better Services for the Mentally Handicapped*. London: HMSO.

Disability Discrimination Act (1995) London: HMSO.

Disability Discrimination Act (2005) London: HMSO.

Education Act (1981) London: HMSO.

Education Act (1993) London: HMSO.

Education (Disability Strategies and Pupils' Educational Records) (Scotland) Act (2002) London: HMSO.

Equalities Act (2010) London: HMSO.

Human Rights Act (1998) London: HMSO.

In Control (2011) 'History of In Control'. [online] Available from http://www.in-control.org.uk/about-us/history-of-in-control.aspx, accessed 11.04.2011.

Inclusive solutions (n.d.) 'What is person centred planning?' [online] Available from http://www.inclusive-solutions.com/pcplanning.asp, accessed 10.04.2011.

Joint Committee on Human Rights (2008) *A Life Like Any Other? Human Rights of Adults with Learning Disabilities* (HL Paper 40-1 HC 73-1). London: HMSO.

Learning Disability Coalition (2007) *Welcome to the learning disability coalition*. [online] Available from http://www.learningdisabilitycoalition.org.uk/download/learning_disability_coalition_easy_read.pdf, accessed 11.04.2011.

Mason, M. (1990) 'Internalised Oppression', in R. Reiser and M. Mason (eds), *Disability Equality in the Classroom: A Human Rights Issue*. London: Inner London Education Authority.

Mencap (2007) *Death by Indifference*. London: Mencap.

Michael Report (2008) *Healthcare for All: Report of the Independent Inquiry into Access to Healthcare for People with Learning Disabilities*. Department of Health: London.

Ministers, local government, NHS, social care, professional and regulatory organisations (2007) *Putting People First: A Shared Vision and Commitment to the Transformation of Adult Social Care*. London: Department of Health.

National Health Service and Community Care Act (1990) London: HMSO.

Oliver, M. (1987) 'Redefining Disability: Some Implications for Research', *Research, Policy and Planning*, 5: 9–13.

Oliver, M. (1990) *The Politics of Disablement*. Tavistock: Macmillan.

Open University (2006a) *Medical Model*. [online] Available from http://www.open. ac.uk/inclusiveteaching/pages/understanding-and-awareness/medical-model.php, accessed 10.04.2011.

Open University (2006b) *Social Model*. [online] Available from http://www.open.ac. uk/inclusiveteaching/pages/understanding-and-awareness/social-model.php, accessed 10.04.2011.

Partners in Policymaking (PiP) (2010) *Partners in Policymaking*. [online] Available from http://www.partnersinpolicymaking.co.uk, accessed 11.04.2011.

Robertson, J., Emerson, E., Hatton, C., Elliott, J., McIntosh, B., Swift, P., Krijnen-Kemp, E., Towers, C., Romeo, R., Knapp, M., Sanderson, H., Routledge, M., Oakes, P. and Joyce, T. (2007) *The Impact of Person Centred Planning for People with Intellectual Disabilities in England: A Summary of Findings*. Lancaster: Institute for Health Research, Lancaster University.

South Gloucestershire Council (2010) *Community Inclusion Champions*. [online] Available from http://www.southglos.gov.uk/NR/exeres/57eb859a-f448-401f-8c36-d6c372491c54, accessed 11.04.2011.

Special Educational Needs and Disability Act (2001). London: HMSO.

United Nations (UN) (2006) *UN Convention on the Rights of Persons with Disabilities*. New York: United Nations General Assembly.

Union of the Physically Impaired Against Segregation (UPIAS) (1976) *Fundamental Principles of Disability*. London: UPIAS.

Warnock Report (1978) *Special Educational Needs*. London: HMSO.

Wolfensberger, W. (1972) *The Principle of Normalization in Human Services*. Toronto: National Institute on Mental Retardation.

Wolfensberger, W. (1998) *A Brief Introduction to Social Role Valorization: A High Order Concept for Addressing the Plight of Socially Devalued People, and for Structuring Human Services*. New York: Syracuse University.

Wolfensberger, W. (2007) *Passing: A Tool for Analyzing Service Quality according to Social Role Valorization Criteria: Ratings Manual*. Syracuse, NY: Training Institute for Human Service Planning, Leadership and Change Agency.

3

ENABLING PEOPLE WITH LEARNING DISABILITIES TO BE VALUED CITIZENS

Sue Hogarth

INTRODUCTION

This chapter will explore the context of citizenship in relation to people with learning disabilities and how people with learning disabilities should be an integral part of their community. Having defined the meaning of citizenship the chapter will discuss the historical evolution of self-advocacy for people with learning disabilities and how this movement has been able to support people to have a voice and implement change locally and nationally. Barriers to citizenship – such as not fully meeting the needs of people with complex learning disabilities and those with a learning disability from black and ethnic minority communities, and producing inaccessible or inappropriate information which hinders understanding – will be explored. Person centred working and person centred planning are pivotal to enabling these changes to take place so the chapter will consider person centred approaches and tools. People with learning disabilities need to be included in planning, monitoring and implementing services for them. This chapter will show how this approach can make a difference for people with learning disabilities and enable them to have a valued and inclusive life. The chapter will conclude with a brief discourse on how employment for people contributes to a full and active life as a citizen.

WHAT IS CITIZENSHIP?

Citizenship is defined in a number of ways. Young Citizens Passport (2006, cited in Owen, 2009) gives us two definitions that are in common use:

A legal and political status: In its simplest meaning, 'citizenship' is used to refer to the status of being a citizen – that is, to being a member of a particular political community or state. Citizenship in this sense brings with it certain rights and responsibilities that are defined in law, such as the right to vote, the responsibility to pay tax and so on. It is sometimes referred to as nationality, and is what is meant when someone talks about 'applying for', 'getting', or being 'refused' citizenship.

Involvement in public life and affairs: The term 'citizenship' is also used to refer to involvement in public life and affairs – that is, to the behaviour and actions of a citizen. It is sometimes known as active citizenship. Citizenship in this sense is applied to a wide range of activities – from voting in elections and standing for political office to taking an interest in politics and current affairs. It refers not only to rights and responsibilities laid down in the law, but also to general forms of behaviour – social and moral – which societies expect of their citizens. What these rights, responsibilities and forms of behaviour should be is an area of ongoing public debate, with people holding a range of views. (Owen, 2009: 1)

The last definition, with its emphasis on the behaviours associated with citizenship and the active processes of citizenship, is closer to how citizenship for people with learning disabilities needs to be understood. Change is about enabling people with learning disabilities to be involved in the process outlined in the definition above but also in the processes that are increasingly being related to the Government's 'Big Society' (Cabinet Office, 2010) with devolved power, local decision making and public participation (DH, 2001a). Breslin et al. refer to:

societies, communities and institutions that promote active citizenship effectively in a range of ways as being 'citizenship-rich'. Citizenship-rich communities are notable for their levels of participation and engagement and are likely to encourage a sense of cohesion and neighbourliness. Indeed, in this sense, many equate being a good citizen with being a good neighbour, demonstrated by showing consideration to others and paying attention to community well being. (2008: 2)

For people with learning disabilities to be enabled to be citizens, there are some specific areas professionals have to consider to ensure people have control over their own lives. Duffy (2010: 262–3) talked about six keys to citizenship:

1 authority – the ability to be in control of your life;

2 direction – having a distinct purpose and meaning to your life;

3 money – having enough resources to direct your own life;

4 home – having a place where you belong;

5 support – needing other people, giving value to the lives of others; and

6 contribution – giving to others through family and community.

Reflection Point 7

When thinking about Duffy's six keys to citizenship, how would the following impact on a person's right to citizenship?

People when they become ill

People who have communication difficulties

People who have literacy problems

People who live in poverty

Are all six keys imperative to full citizenship? What would be the impact if one or more were removed?

If your right to control your life was removed, what impact would this have on your life?

CITIZENSHIP AND LEARNING DISABILITIES

Duffy's citizenship theory (2006) starts from two moral beliefs. First, that all human beings – however different they are in colour, race, gender, body or mind – are fundamentally of equal worth. Second, that human diversity in all forms is a good thing. This fundamental right to be treated as an equal leads us to the principles of his theory. Duffy believes that a fair society is one where everyone is treated with respect and has equal value. This principle asks societies to make a positive definition of citizenship to ensure that those most likely to face discrimination are positively included. He goes on to say that in a fair society members treat each other with mutual respect so that everyone can achieve citizenship and therefore be respected as an equal. For this to happen, society must ensure that everyone gets the right level of support in order for them to achieve citizenship (Duffy, 2010).

SELF-ADVOCACY

When people are unable to speak for themselves, they may have an advocate who speaks and takes actions on their behalf. This is advocacy, sometimes called citizen advocacy. However, self-advocacy is when the person speaks up for themselves and makes things happen (McNally, 2007). McNally talks about advocacy as being fundamental to all people and discusses how, historically, people with a learning disability have had little experience of speaking up for themselves. Self-advocates may therefore need support to be confident and able to speak up and effect real change. The need for such support was met by the development of the self-advocacy movement.

The self-advocacy movement for people with learning disabilities started in Sweden in the 1960s and rapidly spread to North America (Hall, 1999). Various organisations are part of the self-advocacy movement including People First, Speaking for Ourselves, and Self-Advocates Become Empowered (Hall, 1999). In Britain, People First was established in 1984 after a small group of supporters and people with learning disabilities from London went to an international conference on self-advocacy in America. The movement gained momentum with the establishment of People First and Speaking Up groups around the country, initially providing information and telling people with learning disabilities about their rights. The People First self-advocacy movement is a way of uniting people and supporting them to gain control over their own lives. The movement has lagged behind other user-led organisations, such as those for people with a physical disability, due in part to the position of people with learning disabilities in society.

The self-advocacy organisations are clear about the problems people with learning disabilities face in trying to gain more control. One People First group states on its website:

Self-advocacy is people with learning difficulties speaking up for ourselves. Self-advocacy is important because many people with learning difficulties spend their lives being told what to do. If you are always told what to do and never listened to you can get to the point where you don't even know how to make a decision for yourself. Speaking up is something people with learning difficulties need support to learn to do and other people need to learn how to understand us. Self-advocacy has taken forward the idea that people with learning difficulties need to be listened to. Professionals and carers who run services for people with learning difficulties should ask us what we want because no one knows better than us ourselves. (People First)

STRATEGIC PAPERS THAT SUPPORT ADVOCACY AND CITIZENSHIP

Self-advocacy groups have become involved in campaigning to change services through involvement in training staff and as co-researchers. They are also involved in developing government agendas for services for people with learning disabilities. Government departments across Great Britain have become aware of the need to provide services that put people with a learning disability and their carers at the heart of any service. The Scottish Government (2000), Department of Health (2001b), Welsh Assembly Government (2007) and Northern Ireland Assembly (2008) have published their own strategic plans to address the inequalities faced by people who are disadvantaged. Core values in these papers reflect how the new agenda:

> needs to be based on social inclusion, civil rights, choice and independence. People with learning disabilities have the right to be full members of the society in which they live, to choose where they live and what they do, and to be as independent as possible.(DH, 2001b: 21)

The papers have similar principles to those in the Scottish Government paper *The Same as You?*:

- People with learning disabilities should be valued. They should be asked and encouraged to contribute to the community they live in
- They should not be picked on or treated differently from others
- People with learning disabilities are individual people
- People with learning disabilities should be asked about the services they need and be involved in making choices about what they want
- People with learning disabilities should be helped and supported to do everything they are able to
- People with learning disabilities should be able to use the same local services as everyone else, wherever possible
- People with learning disabilities should benefit from specialist social, health and educational services
- People with learning disabilities should have services which take account of their age, abilities and other needs. (2000: 11)

These principles are upheld in *Valuing People* (DH, 2001b):

- Having Legal and Civil Rights
- Supporting Independence
- Having More Choice
- Being Included.

The Scottish Government is committed to policies and strategies that enable people with a learning disability in Scotland to lead full and active lives. Similarly, the Welsh Assembly Government issued a new *Statement on Policy and Practice for Adults with a Learning Disability* in 2007 emphasising the need for people with learning disabilities to have the same rights to citizenship, and to be equal in value and status as all other citizens. Then in January 2008 the Northern Ireland Assembly published *Department of Health, Social Services and Public Safety Equality, Good Relations and Human Rights Strategy and Action Plan,* which detailed the way forward for address-ing the inequalities faced by people who are disadvantaged. It provides a clear direction for services in Northern Ireland, particularly emphasising the need to listen and learn from the experiences of carers and service users in order to address inequalities. People with learning disabilities have been the most isolated and powerless members of society and these strate-gies aim to redress this imbalance supported by legislation such as The Disability Discrimination Act (1995) and Equalities Act (2010) that made it unlawful to discriminate against people in respect of their disabilities.

Reflection Point 8

How could you promote the principles from these policies and strategies in your workplace?

What difficulties might there be in respecting one or more of these principles for service users in your workplace?

What could you do if you felt that people with learning disabilities accessing your services were not supported to have these principles upheld?

One of the ways that *Valuing People* (DH, 2001b) addressed these principles was in the formation of the National Forum in England and its associated Regional Forums. This gave people with learning disabilities the opportu-nity to have a united voice that reported directly to the government. There are nine Regional Forums across England which each elect two representatives to sit on the National Forum. The role of the National Forum is explained on its website (www.nationalforum.co.uk):

> Information is passed on from advocacy groups to regional forums. The regional forums then take this to the National Forum big meeting. The National Forum decides which issues will be passed on to a group called the National Programme Board. This information will then be passed onto Government. The Government will ask us to feedback information and ask what we think about new policies and laws for people with learning difficulties.

Within the forum, the self-advocacy movement has become a national campaigning organisation and they are able to highlight issues facing people with learning disabilities and put them on the national agenda. A good example of this is the work they undertook with government departments about hate crime.

Hate crime against people with learning disabilities is now being taken seriously, with police, the Crown Prosecution Service (CPS) and the judicial system beginning to address the issues of hate crime that people with a learning disability face in their everyday lives. Disability hate crime is now a recognised crime within the judicial system. The law says that people with learning disabilities have the right to protection from Hate Crime (s. 146 of the Criminal Justice Act 2003). The Home Office and Inclusion North describe a Disability Hate Crime as: 'Any criminal offence which is perceived to be motivated because of a person's disability or perceived disability by the victim or any other person' (2008: 2).

The Home Office (2009) launched the *Cross-Government Hate Crime Action Plan*, which includes disability hate crime and addresses the specific issues for people with learning disabilities. This action plan includes some specific commitments around people with learning disabilities, including:

- A review of best practice across the country
- Specific guidance for local Learning Disability Partnership Boards around preventing hate crime incidents, supporting victims and working with other agencies
- A new Crown Prosecution Service policy on prosecuting crimes where people with learning disabilities or mental health problems are victims or witnesses.

Greig (2003) stated that positive change would only happen if there was a local belief in the vision of *Valuing People* (DH, 2001b) and if people were willing to do things differently. People with a learning disability now have a stronger voice and are being listened to by people who can influence change. Although the example above indicates how listening and acting upon concerns can help redress the balance of power, giving people with learning disabilities more control, a report called *Learning Disability Hate Crime: Identifying Barriers to Addressing Crime* (Lamb and Redmond, 2007) showed that it was only happening for a few people. Sustainable change seems harder to achieve.

BARRIERS TO CITIZENSHIP

The report by Greig (2005) used information from *Valuing People* (DH, 2001b) to create a framework for future learning disability services. The report highlighted that there are several challenges to do with choice and control, better lives, and making things happen. The main conclusion of the report was that good practice is patchy and therefore affects few people. People with learning disabilities have faced discrimination for many years and redressing the balance requires a long-term commitment. Greig (2005) highlighted that for people with complex needs or from ethnic minorities little has changed.

People with learning disabilities from black and minority ethnic groups continue to be identified as a particularly discriminated against group (DH, 2009a). This is despite the report commissioned by the Department of Health highlighting the need for a specific focus to be placed on the needs of people from these communities (Mir et al., 2001). The report by Mir et al. (2001) identified the need to engage with ethnic minority communities to ensure that their specific needs are being met and to prevent policies and provision being developed from policy makers' stereotypical views. A person's cultural values and ethnic background are central to their individuality and their role as a citizen. The report also identified the lack of advocacy and self-advocacy organisations that meet the needs of ethnic minority groups. Specialist advocacy organisations were seen as essential in facilitating empowerment of the individual, as they would be able to ensure that the cultural values of the community are recognised. *Valuing People Now* (DH, 2009) has acknowledged that there has not been enough improvement in the involvement of people from black and minority ethnic groups. Part of the new strategy has highlighted the need to work closely with black and minority ethnic groups and has commissioned The National Advisory Group on Learning Disabilities and Ethnicity (NAGLDE) to ensure that the needs of people from these communities are met.

PERSON CENTRED APPROACHES AND CITIZENSHIP

Underpinning strategic papers and reports are the principles of person centred working, including person centred awareness and person centred plans. Person Centred Planning (PCP) started in America and there has been a raft of publications about PCP including Pearpoint et al. (1993), O'Brien and O'Brien (2006, 1998), and Smull et al. (2001). Helen Sanderson Associates define person centred planning as 'a process for continual listening and learning, focussed on what is important to someone now and for the future, and acting upon this in alliance with family and friends'. This listening and learning enables people to understand the person's choices. It requires good communication skills, negotiation and problem solving so that the person's wishes are identified and appropriate support provided to help the individual live their life. Resources may come from existing networks, from service providers and, increasingly, by using personalised budgets to purchase support.

Scenario

I was facilitating a plan for a young man with severe autism, who did not communicate verbally. He invited his hairdresser to his planning meeting. The hairdresser had a unique but effective way of communicating with him that was able to be shared with all the people who supported him in his life. This ranged from paid support workers to members of his local church community.

PCP means putting the person with the learning disability in the centre of planning. The underpinning theory base includes the principles of inclusion and the social model of disability and aims to promote inclusion in their community. It is not just about existing services but also about the possibilities available within their communities and how these can be achieved (DH, 2001c). The process as well as the outcome belongs to the person with learning disabilities, which requires a power shift from those who think they know what the person wants, to actually listening to what the person is saying they want.

Scenario

Andrew is in his 20s and lives with his parents. He did not wish to attend the day centre and was helped to plan alternatives, he plays badminton with one of his circle of support and has successfully climbed the Himalayas after help from his Circle to get fit and join his local Climbing Club. (McIntosh and Whittaker, 1998)

There are a number of tools that can be used to facilitate the person centred plan. These tools are not exclusive, it is the person and how the tools meet their needs that is important. The tools are active ways to identify and record what it is the person wants in their life, how they are going to achieve it and what support they need to be successful. It is a flexible process that sets no limits for the person's wants, needs and dreams for their life. The plan is individual to the person. Plans can be a written document, pictorial representation, PowerPoint presentation, or recorded on a DVD – whichever format is best for the person to own their plan. The person determines the goals and desired outcomes of any plan, with support from their friends, families and staff who are called their circle of support.

There are four main person centred planning tools, each with its own activities and strategies. They are MAPS (Making Action Plans) (Falvey et al., 2000), PATH (Planning Alternative Tomorrows with Hope) (Pearpoint et al., 1993), ELP (Essential Lifestyle Planning) (Smull et al., 2001), and Personal Futures Planning (Mount, 2000). Each tool has its own strengths and does not need to be used exclusively. They can be compared to a tool shed full of gardening tools; you may not need to use all of them at any one time but you do need to know their use so that you can identify which ones you need (Broussine, 2003). The person, with their PCP facilitator and circle of support, decides which tool they will use for their PCP.

For some people it is important to have information about their history and MAPS starts by looking at the person's experiences. This gives an opportunity for people to understand the journey the person has been on. It is particularly useful for people with a learning disability who have been in long-stay institutions and have very little personal history recorded. The MAPS tool also explores nightmares or barriers that stop the person achieving their goals. It explores creative solutions to enable the person to overcome identified barriers.

Scenario

A young woman invited me to her PCP meeting. She has had bouts of depression and anxiety in her past which has impacted on her being able to achieve such things as a trip to New York and paid employment. Developing her MAPS PCP meant she was able to share her anxieties and look at what needed to be put in place to alleviate them. By using this information her circle were able to support her in a way that suited her needs. She used the PATH tool to look at where she was now and she set her goals and targets. She finally achieved a short trip to New York and has held down a part time paid job for a year.

Person centred planning can be used to support everyone to begin to take control of their lives. For people who do not communicate verbally, their circle of support can identify the things that are important to the person as well as what is needed to stay healthy. An Essential Lifestyle Plan provides the framework for this to happen.

TAKING CONTROL

How can supporters and professionals ensure that the balance of power and decision making is shifted so people with learning disabilities have control of their lives? People with learning disabilities have been historically under the control of their parents, carers and professionals. Many professionals still operate within the medical model of disability, seeing the person as being the one with the problem that has to be 'fixed'. Their answers to these perceived problems are seen within the context of professionals who can cure or normalise. There is an understanding that these professionals know best and that their assessments of need are used to determine how people with learning disabilities can lead their lives. While this medical model may have helped to give an understanding of some of the biological causes of learning disability, it has not helped in seeing people as equal citizens who can have full citizenship. Self-advocacy will go some way to redressing this balance because it is based on the concepts of independence, freedom of choice and group awareness.

The People First movement has enabled people with learning disabilities to meet together and share experiences, good and bad. The emergence of the need for people to take hate crime against people with learning disabilities more seriously came about because people with learning disabilities came together at their regional forums to talk about issues which affected them all. During the countrywide consultation prior to *Valuing People Now* (DH, 2009a), local groups identified that relationships were not mentioned anywhere in the document. By working together through their regions and the National Forum, relationships were included in *Valuing People Now*. The work of the National Forum has shown that people with learning disabilities are able to take control and make significant changes in the way they want to live their lives.

Parents, carers and professionals have highlighted their concerns regarding the perceived risks that this independence and choice might involve. In the National Family Carer response to the *Valuing People Now* consultation, some had reservations about people with learning disabilities as local citizens. They were concerned about the safety of their relatives in a 'hostile' community and that independence was only really for the most able

(Cox, 2008). In many areas parents and carers lobbied local MPs when there were plans to close the local day centres. These are seen by many as safe places for their sons and daughters to go. In order for the changes set in the government strategy document to happen professionals need to rethink their way of working and become enablers not only for people with learning disabilities but for parents and carers too. There are examples of shifts in the power base, with people with learning disabilities becoming involved in staff recruitment, training and in the monitoring of service quality.

Recruiting Staff

People with learning disabilities are becoming more involved in the recruiting of staff. A good example of this is where people with learning disabilities are involved in the whole recruitment process, not just the interviewing of staff. Job descriptions and person specifications are written in easy read. The shortlisting process is done jointly with the person with a learning disability who, having independent support if necessary, has an equal say in that process. Interview questions are devised jointly and in the final decision as to appointment the person with a learning disability again has an equal say. There were initial concerns raised about whether they would choose the most suitable candidate but these concerns were not borne out. As long as the person had the appropriate training and the information was accessible, decisions on appointment of staff have been agreed by all parties.

Training Staff

People with learning disabilities are also being more involved in training. This makes sense as they are the experts and know from first-hand knowledge what staff need to be doing. Many organisations – including service providers and universities – are involving people in both formal and informal learning activities. This works very well when people with learning disabilities co-teach with others with whom they have developed empowering ways of working and where the value of both trainers is seen as equal. Understanding and meeting individuals' support needs so they can be active and successful trainers is good for the individuals, the organisation employing them and the learners (Owen et al., 2004).

Quality Inspector

The need for people with learning disabilities to be involved in evaluating the quality of services is now being recognised, with organisations such as

CQC employing people with learning disabilities to be part of the inspection process in residential homes. People are realising that people with learning disabilities are the best people to check the quality of provision. They have experienced these types of provision and, as such, are 'Experts by Experience'. The Commission for Social Care Inspection (CSCI), now the Care Quality Commission, produced a leaflet detailing the benefits of involving people who use services in their inspections (CSCI, 2008). This model is now being used by many authorities across England to check on the quality of services being provided for people with a learning disability.

EMPLOYMENT

One of the most important activities to becoming an active citizen in the local community is being able to have a worthwhile paid job. Employment plays an enormous role in all of our lives. Financially we are better off, but it is the value-added aspects of employment that are most important. Where do you meet most of your friends? What dominates a lot of your conversation? How many times do you say 'Can't be too late tonight as I have to go to work tomorrow' or 'Thank goodness it is only five days to pay day'? This is an area that the majority of people with learning disabilities are excluded from.

Scenario

Some members of a self-advocacy group went to talk to their local council. They talked about the skills they had, the numerous work experience placements they had been on, the plethora of certificates they had obtained from the local college and the fact that they could not get a paid job at the end of all this. They were able to point out that the local council were the biggest employer in the area and asked them how many people with learning disabilities they employed. After much nervous debate the answer was 'Two', to which the self-advocates replied 'What are you going to do about it'. This led to the council re-looking at its recruitment process, investigating the Mencap Workright programme and starting to look at the possibility of job carving.

They have not got it right yet but at least it is a step in the right direction. Within the scheme, managers of each department need to be champions who can be more creative about how they see job roles and recruitment.

Valuing Employment Now (DH, 2009b) states that one in five jobs in Britain are in the public sector, but employment of people with disabilities in the public sector is lower than in the rest of the economy (Hirst et al., 2004). *Valuing Employment Now* sets targets for increasing work opportunities for people with learning disabilities supported by funding for job coaching through existing funding streams such as personal budgets.

Reflection Point 9

Do you see employees with learning disabilities in your workplace? If your answer is yes then you are in a minority. However if your answer is no what do you think this says about how inclusive your working environment is? If you are not involved in the employment of staff, you could bring it up at a staff meeting in order to identify and discuss the prejudices and bias people have against employment of people with disabilities. Bringing this topic into the open starts to raise awareness, which is the beginning of effecting change.

There are many preconceived ideas about employing people with a learning disability, including health and safety issues, a lack of awareness about available support and not knowing how to work with someone with learning disabilities. The scenario below mentions job carving, which entails identifying aspects of a job that a person with learning disabilities can do and having this as a real, paid job (DH, 2009b).

Scenario

Adam studied at UWE and loved the library. He wanted to work there. Adam's mum encouraged him to volunteer. The library staff were enthusiastic and identified a work activity that Adam could do (job carved one task from the library assistant job description). With advice from Mencap, employment systems were adapted and Adam started volunteering tagging library resources. Adam loved working in the library and successfully applied for a job. The library staff feel that having Adam working in the Library is important as often 'social inclusion' and 'equality and diversity' are only talked about, but this is about making work a reality for Adam. Adam has had a profound effect on the people with whom he works, he is clever and very able, and quite the comic at times. (Adapted from an article in *Involved*, University of West England, 2011)

Many people with a learning disability want a paid job, but despite efforts to provide training, qualifications and work experience people are usually unemployed (DH, 2009b).

CONCLUSION

While no one would argue that full citizenship is not a right for people with a learning disability, achieving this right is far more complex. Historically people with a learning disability have been seen, at best, as needing care and, at worst, as having no rights. There have been many guidance documents from governments and assemblies across the UK since 2000 but there is still a long way to go before people achieve equal citizenship. People from black and ethnic minority groups who have a learning disability are more disadvantaged and the advocacy movement ability to provide support for people from ethnic minority groups has been slow to emerge. Person centred ways of working are key to ensuring that the voices of people with learning disabilities are at the heart of any work or service delivery. A more creative approach to providing services needs to be embedded, where the people using the services are seen as equal citizens. This will become more of a reality with the emergence of personal budgets, where people with a learning disability will buy the services that they have identified will best suit them. People with learning disabilities are becoming aware of their right to be an integral part of their community. Their aspirations are high and individuals are asking why they cannot have the same opportunities as anyone else. By using the social model of disability, people are starting to explore how individuals with learning disabilities can become equal citizens. The challenge for everyone is to start from the premise that we are all equal citizens and then ensure that the right support is provided to enable people with learning disabilities to be valued as equals.

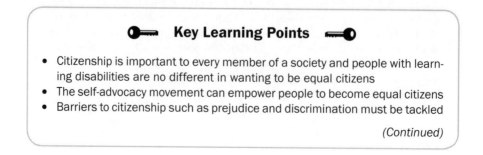

⚷ Key Learning Points ⚷

- Citizenship is important to every member of a society and people with learning disabilities are no different in wanting to be equal citizens
- The self-advocacy movement can empower people to become equal citizens
- Barriers to citizenship such as prejudice and discrimination must be tackled

(Continued)

- Person centred ways of working are central to supporting individuals to live a full life
- Employment is important and people with learning disabilities make good employees. Employment provides wages, opportunities for friendships and status, thus promoting equal citizenship.

REFERENCES

Breslin, T., Cavanaugh, C., Ellis, D., Green, S., Harwood, N., Huddleston, T., Raeburn, D., Ratiu, R., Sofola, A. and Thornton, A. (2008) *Exploring Citizenship. Building Participation: Initial Submission to the Youth Citizenship Commission.* [online] Available from http://www.citizenshipfoundation.org.uk/lib_res_pdf/0785.pdf, accessed 09.04.2011.

Broussine, E. (2003) 'Being flexible with PCP tools to meet individuals' needs', Lecture Notes: Person Centred Planning. Bristol: University of the West of England.

Cabinet Office (2010) *Building a Big Society.* [online] Available from http://www.cabinetoffice.gov.uk/sites/default/files/resources/building-big-society_0.pdf, accessed 09.04.2011.

Cox, J. (2008) *Response To Valuing People Now Consultation.* Bristol: National Family Carer Network.

Criminal Justice Act (2003). London: HMSO.

The Commission for Social Care Inspection (CSCI) (2008) *Experts by Experience. The Benefits of Experience: Involving People Who use Services in Inspections.* London: The Commission for Social Care Inspection.

Department of Health (2001a) *Public participation methods: evolving and operationalising an evaluation framework – developing and testing a toolkit for evaluating the success of public participation exercises summary project report.* London: Department of Health.

Department of Health (2001b) *Valuing People: A New Strategy for Learning Disability for the 21st Century.* London: Department of Health.

Department of Health (2001c) *Towards Person Centred Approaches: Guidance for Implementation Groups.* London: Department of Health.

Department of Health (2009a) *Valuing People Now: A New Three Year Strategy for People with Learning Disabilities.* London: Department of Health.

Department of Health (2009b) *Valuing Employment Now: Real Jobs for People with Learning Disabilities.* London, Department of Health.

Disability Discrimination Act (1995). London: HMSO.

Duffy, S. (2006) *Keys to Citizenship.* Liverpool: Paradigm.

Duffy, S. (2010) 'The Citizenship Theory of social justice: exploring the meaning of personalisation for social workers', *Journal of Social Work Practice,* 24 (3): 253–67.

Equalities Act (2010) London: HMSO.

Falvey, M., Forest, M., Pearpoint, J. and Rosenberg, R. (2000) *All My Life's a Circle – Using the Tools: Circles, MAPs and PATH.* Toronto: Inclusion Press.

Greig, R. (2003) 'Changing the culture', *British Journal of Learning Disabilities*, 31: 151–2.

Grieg, R. (2005) *Valuing People. The Story So Far … A New Strategy for Learning Disability for the 21st Century*. London: Department of Health.

Hall, M. (1999). *NRC Fact Sheet: What is Self-Advocacy?* Syracuse, NY: National Resource Center on Supported Living and Choice, Center on Human Policy.

Helen Sanderson Associates (n.d.) *Person Centred Planning*. [online] Available from http://www.helensandersonassociates.co.uk/what-we-do/how/person-centred-planning.aspx, accessed 09.04.2011.

Hirst, M., Thornton, P. and Dearey, M. (2004) *The Employment of Disabled People in the Public Sector: A Review of Data and Literature*. London: Disabilities Rights Commission.

Home Office (2009) *Hate Crime – The Cross-government Action Plan*. [online] Available from http://www.arcsafety.net/page7/assets/Hate%20Crime%20Good%20Practice%20 Guide.pdf, accessed 10.04.2011.

Home Office and Inclusion North (2008) *Learning Disability Hate Crime: Good Practice Guidance for Crime and Disorder Reduction*. London: Home Office and Inclusion North.

Lamb, L., Redmond, M. (2007) *Learning Disability Hate Crime: Identifying Barriers to Addressing Crime*. London: Care Services Improvement Partnership, Valuing People Support Team.

McIntosh, B. and Whittaker, A. (1998) *Days of Change: A Practical Guide to Developing Better Day Opportunities with People with Learning Disabilities*. London: Kings Fund.

McNally, S. (2007) 'Helping to Empower People', in B. Gates (ed.), *Learning Disabilities: Towards Inclusion* (5th edn). Edinburgh: Churchill Livingstone.

Mencap (n.d.) *Jobs and Training*. [online] Available from http://www.mencap.org.uk/ page.asp?id=13714, accessed 10.04.2011.

Mir, G., Nocon, A., Ahmad, W. and Jones, L. (2001) *Learning difficulties and Ethnicity Report to the Department of Health*. London: Department of Health.

Mount, B. (2000) *Life Building. Opening Windows to Change: Using Personal Futures Planning Personal Workbook*. New York: Capacity Works.

Northern Ireland Assembly (2008) *Department of Health, Social Services and Public Safety Equality, Good Relations and Human Rights Strategy and Action Plan*. Belfast: Department of Health, Social Service and Public Safety.

O'Brien, J. and O'Brien, C.L. (1998) *A Little Book about Person Centred Planning*. Toronto: Inclusion Press.

O'Brien, J. and O'Brien, C.L. (2006) *Implementing Person Centred Planning: Voices of Experience*. Toronto: Inclusion Press.

Owen, C. (2009) *Issues Today: Citizenship and Identity* (issue 32). Cambridge: Independence Educational Publishers.

Owen, K., Butler, G. and Hollins, S. (2004) *A New Kind of Trainer: How to Develop the Training Role for People with Learning Disabilities*. London: Gaskell.

Pearpoint, J., O'Brien, J., and Forest, M. (1993) *PATH (Planning Alternative Tomorrows with Hope): A Workbook for Planning Positive Futures*. Toronto: Inclusion Press.

People First *What is Self Advocacy?* [website] Available from http://www.peoplefirstltd. com/what-is-self-advocacy.php, accessed on 09.04.2011.

Scottish Government (2000) *The Same as You? A Review of Services for People with Learning Disabilities*. Edinburgh: The Scottish Government.

Smull, M., Sanderson, H. and Allen, B. (2001) *Essential Lifestyle Planning: A Handbook for Facilitators*. Manchester: Northwest Training and Development Team.

University of the West of England (2011) 'Adam Progresses From Student, To Volunteer To Employee', *Involved*, 12. [online] Available from http://hls.uwe.ac.uk/suci/Data/Sites/1/issue12.pdf, accessed 10.04.2011.

Welsh Assembly Government (2007) *Statement on Policy and Practice for Adults with a Learning Disability*. Cardiff: Welsh Assembly Government.

4 LIVING WITH A LEARNING DISABILITY

Dawn Rooke and Kim Scarborough

INTRODUCTION

The UK government has an ambition that all people will live full lives that promote dignity, well-being and independence (DH, 2007a). It is important for health and social care professionals to use person centred thinking if this is going to happen and people with learning disabilities are truly to be treated with dignity and have full lives (Robertson et al., 2005). To be person centred professionals need an awareness of the lives of people with learning disabilities and their families in order to ask useful questions and respond in helpful ways. This chapter offers an exploration of the lives of people with learning disabilities and their families throughout the life continuum. Starting with finding out that your child has a learning disability and moving through the main life stages of pre-school, school age, transition to adult service, adulthood and older people. Throughout these stages support for carers is important and so there is a brief discussion on meeting the needs of carers towards the end of the chapter. The chapter aims to provide an insight into the lived experiences of people, enabling the professional to recognise the different life experiences that some people may have had and to understand the need to be positive in their interactions with people with learning disabilities and their family carers.

SO WHAT DOES A FULL LIFE LOOK LIKE?

While this will vary for different individuals, the common theme is that – whatever our age – having friends, families and relationships are important. *Valuing People* (DH, 2001) acknowledged how socially isolated people with learning disabilities can be and how challenging it is to reduce social isolation. Members of the South Gloucestershire Community Champions (SGCC), a group of adults with learning disabilities who promote inclusion, spoke about what makes their lives good:

'My mum and brothers are the most important people in my life'

'I love living in my own flat with my husband'

'I have friends from the old day centre; we meet up to do things together'

'Having personal assistants that I can trust is important'

'Working with people I like makes me very happy'.

However ordinary these statements may seem, many people with learning disabilities need support to maintain these relationships and develop new ones. Support might include the active participation of paid carers in providing physical opportunities to meet with family or friends. It may be helping someone use public transport and communication technologies, such as the internet and telephones. It might involve using specialist communication devices and aids such as picture boards and communication passports to ensure people can communicate effectively. It certainly involves listening to what the individual person wants from their lives. Chapters 6 and 7 focus on relationships and communication so we do not propose to explore them here, but what is written in this chapter needs to be considered in the context of people who have learning disabilities and their families placing high value on positive relationships and good communication as a basis for actions that promote full lives.

HAVING A CHILD WITH A LEARNING DISABILITY

Scenario

Dawn's experiences. As a parent of three children, two of whom have learning disabilities, I can tell you there is a swift learning curve. When you are faced

(Continued)

(Continued)

with the unexpected problems that having a child with learning disabilities can bring it can seem devastating. Having had one son I realised that my second son was experiencing problems communicating, interacting and socialising. Then my third son had similar problems and I realised I needed expert help. Both my sons were referred to a paediatrician. My youngest son was diagnosed aged four with 'Autistic Tendencies'. However, my other son was more of a 'patchwork quilt' of differences and went from 'Severe Language Disorder' aged two, then 'Aspergers Syndrome' aged seven, to 'Autistic Spectrum Disorder' aged 17. Our family had a lot of input from the Community Learning Disabilities Team (CLDT), paediatrics, psychiatry and staff at the children's special school. Much of my support, as a parent, came from other families in a similar position – sharing stories and strategies and learning from each other. Sharing experiences helped each of us understand the problems faced and possible solutions. Having people direct us to these support networks was important in helping us feel we were not alone, or mad, and the real experts – other parents – were able to help us understand and truly enjoy our lives with our children.

Dawn's story reflects findings from Mencap (n.d.) when she talks about feelings of devastation when parents find out they have a child with learning disabilities; she also clearly demonstrates that finding this out can take a long time and diagnosis is not always a simple task. This in itself brings stress and anxiety, often associated with contact with so many professionals (Scarborough, 2005). However, Dawn ends with how other parents have helped her understand her life with her children. Good support from other parents can help new parents recognise that parenting a child with learning disabilities may bring additional stressors but it is rewarding and, in so many ways, the same as parenting any child. It is important that professionals are able to direct parents to informal support systems. Dawn talks about the help she received from services and it is important that professionals direct parents and carers to high quality information about what services are available. The Childcare Act (2006) led to the implementation in April 2008 of the statutory duty for all local services to provide information, in ways parents can understand, until a child is 20 years of age (Department for Children, Schools and Families [DCSF], 2006). Knowing where services are and where information is held should be a priority for any professionals working with parents who have a child with learning disabilities, or a parent who has a learning disability (Department of Health and Department for Education and Skills, 2007).

> ### Reflection Point 10
>
> Are you aware of the help available for parents who have a child with learning disabilities? How do you contact your local Learning Disability Specialist Services and how do you make a referral? What support groups exist in your area? Next time you are using the internet take ten minutes to gather some basic information about your local services.

PRE-SCHOOL CHILDREN

Most parents will initially go to their GP or health visitor for advice and support. These professionals manage initial concerns and refer to other services as appropriate and, with learning disabilities nurses integrated into children's services, joint working can improve access to specialist services. Parents of pre-school children with learning disabilities, as Mencap (n.d.) notes, have the same issues as all parents. Issues such as finding childcare, choosing the right school, managing health and toilet training can be more complex because of the specific needs of individual children. Mencap (n.d.) also lists the more specific systems that families have to engage with, including obtaining statutory assessments to ensure appropriate support systems are available and building relationships with professionals. There is a range of services available designed to provide support for parents and carers such as Sure Start (visit www.education.gov.uk), which provides advice on child health, parenting and specialist services (Directgov, 2011). There is also PORTAGE, a pre-school home visiting programme that parents of children with learning disabilities can access. The PORTAGE visitors can provide advice, support and training to maximise both the child's and the family's quality of life (visit http://www.portage.org.uk/index.php). Support from other parents while learning how to work within professionally led systems is essential. Dawn notes how it made her feel she was not alone.

GOING TO SCHOOL AND CHILDHOOD

Today, most children with learning disabilities will receive mainstream education, meaning education at the local school with non-disabled peers. To receive additional support in a mainstream school, or to be able to attend a special school, the child is assessed and a statement of needs is written (Special Educational Needs and Disability Act 2001). Dawn mentions that her sons went to a special school. These schools provide specialist education for people with a range of needs. For children with learning disabilities this would include the existence of a learning disability, but children might also have additional physical or sensory impairments or emotional or mental health needs. Many special schools have strong links with local mainstream schools with children participating in joint learning activities. While mainstream education is an expectation for many families of children with learning disabilities, it is not trouble free. Children with learning disabilities are twice as likely to be bullied as other children (Mencap, 2007). This increased risk of bullying has led to government guidelines aimed at tackling these anti-social and damaging behaviours in schools and children's services (Department for Children, Schools and Families, 2008).

Children with learning disabilities need friends with similar life experiences as themselves, alongside non-disabled friends within their communities. Cook et al. (2001) point out that being with other children with similar impairments provides positive personal and social outcomes and that it is important that the experiences of having an impairment are acknowledged as part of who the child is. This is not about advocating for segregated education or leisure for disabled children. Cook et al. (2001) also found that children with impairments who had inclusive education had a strong feeling of belonging to their community and responded well to the increased expectations that mainstream education presents.

Due to higher health needs, children and young people with learning disabilities have frequent contact with health services. This means services have to become accessible and ensure equality regarding outcomes. Child and Adolescent Mental Health services (CAMHs) have had to consider how they will meet the needs of those who have a learning disability and the Foundation of People with Learning Disabilities (2006) has worked with children, young people and their families to develop guidelines out-lining good practice in CAMH services. These guidelines include improvements in referral systems, thinking more about the environment where people are seen and how inviting it is or stigmatising, develop-ments in accessible information, and improvements in how professionals work together.

MOVING FROM CHILD TO ADULT SERVICES

When people move from child to adult services it is a major life transition. Young people with learning disabilities have a right to an education until the age of 19, however, transition planning starts at age 13–14 and can continue until age 25. *Valuing People Now* (DH, 2009a) states that the director of social services is responsible for ensuring adult and child services have strong links, making transitions easier. On a more personal level Connexions Services or the local authority should provide personal advisers to help children and their families plan for the future, developing person centred plans for continued education, day activities or employment and health action plans to optimise communication between adult and child health services (DH, 2009a). However, transition planning is often lacking due to young people receiving poor coordination of transfers to adult services. It is good practice for local authorities to develop their partnership approach to transition planning and have a single contact person to ensure a person centred process which supports a smooth transfer from child to adult services for disabled young people (DH, 2007b).

Scenario

Dawn's experiences. Approaching Transition can be very stressful. The complexity of the benefits system as well as considering the options of work, training, and employment can all add to stress levels, raising anxiety, but knowing your young person really well helps to keep anxiety levels down. Using the person centred approaches introduced in Chapter 3 and being able to gather detailed, vital information on what is important to my son and how to support him has changed all our family's lives. Helping young people belong to their communities is a huge part of ensuring they live a full and happy life. My son looks forward to his excursions and his behaviour has improved. This is due to selecting appropriate staff, with excellent training in Autism, who understand how to manage his anxieties.

Ensuring the correct and most suitable provision for the young person is very difficult. Developing a unified approach to Transition has helped families and professionals be clear about what is expected from them. Parent handbooks have helped families know what they are entitled to, enabling families to question authorities if they do not receive the relevant help, a good example being *My Transition: Guide for Parents, Professionals and Partnership Services* (Highland Council, 2008). In addition, the Gloucestershire Multi Agency Transition Group (2011) has developed a 'Transition Pathway' as a result of funding from Every Disabled Child Matters, to assist families. All agencies have signed up to a single person centred process to allow a smooth transfer from child to adult services for those young people who have had an education statement.

Transition planning requires active listening to find out what the young person wants and working in ways that will help them make decisions about their lives. Empowering young people and their families helps develop a better future; many individuals just want the same as their peers – to work, to go out with friends and to have a life.

ADULTS WITH LEARNING DISABILITIES

Adults with learning disabilities can and do live full lives. They exercise their right to get married, have children, vote and be part of society. Full citizenship discussed in the previous chapter alongside person centred ways of working with people can help support people to live the life they want. When this works people are supported to live with whom they want, to have a job, and to access the facilities and services that are available to all citizens.

Scenario

Charlie had spent many years living in an institution. When the institution was being closed he left and lived for a few years in a care home but did not like it much. He wanted his own place with his friend and he wanted to be a bus driver. Most people told him he was being unrealistic but Charlie never let go of his dream. One day his care manager asked him what he wanted in his life. He told his dream of having a flat and being a bus driver. This time someone listened. The care manager found out from Charlie that the important thing about being a bus driver was working with the buses, having a uniform and chatting with the drivers. With support, Charlie found a job cleaning the buses at the local bus depot. He had a uniform with the bus company logo on and a pass to the staff canteen where he could chat with the bus drivers. About a year later he moved into his own flat with his friend and with appropriate support lived independently. Charlie said that his dreams had come true, he was not a bus driver but what he did have through his work at the depot was sufficient to make him happy. The core of his dream was achievable, but only when someone listened.

Unfortunately good support is not always available. An example is parenthood. Parents with learning disabilities can and do make good parents (see Working Together with Parents Network and Norah Fry, 2009) but require support to be competent parents; however, this is often not forthcoming. Therefore a parent with a learning disability is at much higher risk of having their child removed from their care, indeed Emerson et al. (2005)

found that 48 per cent of the parents with learning disabilities that they interviewed were not living with their children. Good practice guides to support those who work with parents who have a learning disability have been developed (see Department of Health and Department for Education and Skills, 2007) but the most important theme is that a parent's incompetence must not be assumed.

Many people with learning disabilities continue to live in the family home with their parents or siblings. Where people with learning disabilities continue living at home, it is sometimes the person with a learning disability who becomes the carer as they take on the responsibility for caring for their ageing parents or their partner. When this happens their caring role is often not acknowledged, meaning they do not get the support they are entitled to (DH, 2009a). Accessing information on the support that carers can ask for can be difficult for someone who has learning disabilities, as a carer who has a learning disability may need support to complete forms.

ADULT EDUCATION, OCCUPATION AND WORK

Government policy for the modernisation of specialist day services for people with learning disabilities has involved the closure of traditional services and the growth of individualised services including employment, further education, leisure, time at home and socialising with friends (Valuing People Support Team, 2004). People with learning disabilities and their families often experience anxiety as their lives change when moving from centralised service provision to individualised support. A South Gloucestershire Community Champion said about his day service closing, 'My mum is worried. But we think it is scary. But it will be OK. People were scared when [institution] closed but it was good, this will be good too'. Such service changes are enabling more community inclusion, independence and less reliance on families. However, change should not reduce opportunities for people with learning disabilities to develop and maintain friendships with their peers but enrich lives by supporting people to form additional new friendships.

Work helps people with learning disabilities feel good about themselves (Mencap, 2009), but it can be difficult to find a job (DH, 2009b). Despite an emphasis on work in both *Valuing People* (DH, 2001) and *Valuing People Now* (DH, 2009a), people with learning disabilities experience high unemployment rates (Foster, 2009). Anne McGuire, the minister for disabled people in 2005, noted how 'the 90 per cent unemployment rate among people with a learning disability remains a huge inequality in our society'

(O'Bryan and Beyer, 2005: 2). When compared to the unemployment rate of 8 per cent for the general population in 2011 (Office of National Statistics, 2011) the inequality is stark. In the UK disabled people can access support to improve employment prospects through the Work Choice Programme (Department for Work and Pensions [DWP], 2010). This programme provides mentoring, work skills and supports employers – making success a real possibility. The *Real Lives, Real Talent, Real Jobs* (HM Government and DH, 2010) programme provides a range of examples of how to help people with learning disabilities gain employment. These include job coaching, which entails working with employers to reduce negative attitudes and overcome perceived barriers to employment, and working with the individual person with learning disabilities to help them learn how to work and develop their confidence and self-esteem. To support people into employment some employers also participate in job carving. This entails identifying aspects of a role that a person with learning disabilities would be able to do and advertising this as a job. For some individuals volunteering can provide opportunities to develop both networks and work skills. However, until an individual finds a paid job they need to understand how to maximise their income, be it through benefits or access to other forms of grant. The development of a Transition Plan or Person Centred Plan can help when trying to support an individual to gain employment as such a plan includes all the interests of that person and can give helpful clues as to the strengths they have which can be utilised.

Adult education opportunities can help people into paid employment. Computer skills, literacy, numeracy and preparation for work are topics studied. Also NVQ levels 1 and 2 are studied in a range of work areas including childcare, catering and customer service. Where these courses are studied at college with work experience built in, people with learning disabilities are able to participate in work life gaining valuable training and possibly a job or a reference. The value of adult education opportunities is felt not only by people with learning disabilities but also by carers.

Scenarios

Dawn's experiences.   Having three individuals with disabilities in our house, it has been almost impossible for me to work. However, I was not prepared to just sit back and let caring be my life. I decided that to ensure the best possible future for my children, I needed to understand the processes they would go through and discover the best ways in which this could be done. I embarked on educating myself and started studying for a Certificate in Higher Education at the University of the West of England, which explored Person Centred Planning. Working in a person centred way was all I'd ever known with my children and I consumed the information with relish. Alongside this I started doing Health and Social Care subjects with the Open University, as well as attending meetings as a carer representative. After a long but determined struggle I gained my Degree in December 2008. I feel I have used my time in a positive way as I am now in a position to look at re-entering the work arena.

Leisure and Social Lives

Enjoying leisure time is important for all of us and how people with learning disabilities spend their leisure time is as diverse as any sector of the population. Leisure activities might be focussed around the television or computer. Also leisure might need to be supported with accessible written materials; either talking books, or books in Braille, or accessible instructions or forms. Accessing leisure activities out of the home does present a number of barriers. Beart (2001) notes how people need practical support. Few people with learning disabilities drive so having access to appropriate transport is essential. As already discussed, people with learning disabilities may not have a paid job and so poverty might be a significant barrier to accessing leisure services like sports facilities or venues, restaurants, public houses and entertainment venues. Also, the attitudes of staff and the public can be a barrier.

Meeting up with friends and family is important for people, as is finding opportunities to meet new friends. People with learning disabilities are setting up their own friendship and dating groups. An example is the Stars in the Sky (2005) group that was established in London in 2005 and now has six branches. These groups offer opportunities for people with learning disabilities to maintain relationships and develop new ones. They also pro-vide information on staying safe, sex and relationships and can support people to access appropriate advice on contraception and domestic violence.

The Right Home and Most Appropriate Support – Leaving Home

Mencap (2009) states that people with learning disabilities need choice about where they live and need to be supported to find the place they feel is right for them. For this to happen throughout an individual's life choices need to be offered as they age. People need to be able to stay at home or go to residential schools/colleges during both compulsory and post-compulsory education. They need choice in how short breaks are taken. They need choice when it is time for them to leave the family home and again if their needs change, for example due to increased skills and confidence, new relationships or health changes (Mencap, 2009).

People with learning disabilities and their family carers have a range of options for managing their accommodation and care. Some people with learning disabilities will remain in the family home for most, if not all of their lives. Their parents or siblings will be their main carers and take on the coordination of a wide range of services (Scarborough, 2005). Residential or nursing care homes provide communal living that meets individual needs; however, there is a move towards supported living. This offers more individualised care packages with more choice on types of accommodation and who people live with. For people who have complex needs there is a growing number of Family Trusts developing which manage budgets, employ staff and provide individualised care (Clarke et al., 2007). The personalisation agenda has supported changes in how health budgets, social care monies, personal budgets, independent living allowances, housing allowances and mobility allowances are accessed and used.

Reflection Point 11

Are you aware that families and people with learning disabilities are increasingly managing their own budgets? These budgets might consist of benefits and grants from a range of sources. This means people are empowered to employ their own staff. What do you think the issues might be for a person with learning disabilities who employs their own staff? If you were providing healthcare to a person with learning disabilities how might you either support their staff in developing good practice or challenge bad practice? What is your role if you felt the staff were taking advantage of a vulnerable adult? Check your policies and procedures if you are not sure about your role in reporting suspected abuse or neglect.

OLDER PEOPLE WITH LEARNING DISABILITIES

People with learning disabilities are benefiting from improvements in healthcare and advances in medicine resulting in many living into old age. Also, becoming older does not necessarily relate to having a poorer quality of life (Scope, 2007), indeed McCausland et al. (2008) found that if individuals had employment they often wanted to continue working past retirement age. Where the individual is living in residential care or supported living, many homes now aim to provide care into old age and often those who monitor the home allow this to happen and do not expect people to move out of their home and go into a home for older people. Wilkinson et al. (2004) call this 'ageing in place' and consider it good practice.

As people with learning disabilities age they develop the same health problems as all people (Hollins et al., 1998). However, healthcare staff are unprepared for meeting these people's needs (Michael, 2008). In addition to normal aging processes people with learning disabilities have a higher risk of developing dementia and for some people, especially those with Down's syndrome, dementia can develop at an earlier age than in the general population and be difficult to diagnose (Strydom and Hassiotis, 2003). As dementia is discussed later in this book the point to make here is that caring for a 55-year-old son or daughter with dementia when the carers are themselves 75 years of age or over brings many additional stresses meaning respite care is very important.

POVERTY AND PEOPLE WITH LEARNING DISABILITIES AND THEIR FAMILIES

Historically, families of individuals who have complex needs – for example those with behaviours that are difficult to manage, or individuals with high health needs or profound learning disabilities – have had to face varying degrees of financial constraint. Poverty contributes to high risk of ill health and lower achievements (Department for Children, Schools and Families, 2003). Lack of opportunity for individuals and their carers to work, lack of access to support or limited services being available due to eligibility criteria, can all have a huge impact on how a family manages financially (Mencap, 2001). Accessing benefits also relies on the availability of information about the individual's and family's entitlements and the ability to complete complex forms. Offering benefit advice is complex due to regular changes to benefit entitlement. It is better to refer people to the Department for Work and Pensions or the Citizens Advice Bureau or Carer Centre rather than trying to give information that might be inaccurate. With advice likely to be complex, supporting the individual either by going with them or by recommending they go with an advocate or support worker is essential.

CARE FOR CARERS

Some families have a range of professionals involved in their lives. Preventing stress to families is very important as it will help them maintain their ability to be able to cope better when dealing with the everyday problems they face when trying to ensure their child has the best quality of life possible. In order to ensure a carer can continue to provide care, the statutory services need to carry out a carer's assessment to establish the needs of that carer under the Carers Act (1995) and the Carers and Disabled Children Act (2000). To ensure that the carer receives the support they need it is important they receive a carer assessment to identify whether they can manage or whether some input is necessary to maintain their health and well-being, and to ensure carers are identified by their local authorities (Carers UK, 2010). The government guidance document – *Carers at the Heart of the 21st Century Families and Communities: A Caring System on Your Side, A Life of Your Own* (DH, 2008) – highlights the need for carers to have the same access to the outside world as others not in a caring role. To enable this to happen, authorities need to put a system in place that provides adequate support for the cared for, so if the need is that the carer wants to go to work, they can do so without worrying.

SHORT BREAKS

Short breaks give parents and carers time to do other things, especially time to rest and spend time with other family members, including other children. The individual who receives the short-break should also benefit from experiences they might not otherwise have. However, the *Breaking Point* report from Mencap (2006) identified that short breaks were still not being offered, with families struggling to manage. Mencap define breaking point as:

> a physical and emotional crisis, where the persistent lack of short break services and the endless pressure of providing intensive care finally take their toll. It is a dreadful situation for families, which causes pain and despair and, often, irreparable damage. (2006: 5)

In order to prevent people reaching breaking point there needs to be support in place which enables carers to care for themselves, for other family members and to do the ordinary life things that being a carer interrupts. Sixty per cent of carers reported ill health due to the amount of care they needed to provide (Mencap, 2006). Mencap's *Breaking Point* report focussed on carers of people with profound learning disabilities and found that, on average, carers provided fifteen hours' care a day with disturbed nights seven days a week. However, with good support, people need not reach breaking point. Short breaks are provided in a number of ways. Some people have paid support in their home allowing families to have time away from providing care. For some people shared care in another family means the person with learning disabilities is not in the family home but remains in a family situation. There is also residential provision where people with learning disabilities stay in a facility which provides an appropriate level of care and support for small groups of people. When people have life-limiting illnesses they might access hospice care either in their own home or at a hospice. Mencap (2006) reports that only 1 in 13 children and 1 in 5 adults (who receive services) have short breaks, with insufficient resources, lack of provision and choice contributing to the problems.

Reflection Point 12

List the things you do in an average workday, day off, week, month, year. You will probably include meeting colleagues, swimming, shopping, holidays, family get togethers, etc. When you have completed your list spend a little time noting how being a 24-hour carer for a family member could impact on your ordinary life. What support do you think you would need to maintain some ordinariness in your life?

CONCLUSION

Many family carers provide care from when their child is born until either they or their child dies. Even if their son or daughter leaves home they often provide the constant source of support and advocacy that ensures the person has the ordinary life they want. Although people with learning disabilities have historically had very different lives to many people in their community this is changing. Integration into mainstream education, inclusion in work and participation in local leisure activities are making people with learning disabilities visible in their communities. This is not without its difficulties, and prejudice and even hate crime exist. But people are striving to be members of their community and have ordinary lives. Having learning disabilities does present challenges that may be exacerbated when individuals are treated as unequal citizens and when their rights are undermined, but people with learning disabilities and their families are as capable of having an ordinary family life as any other person with the right support.

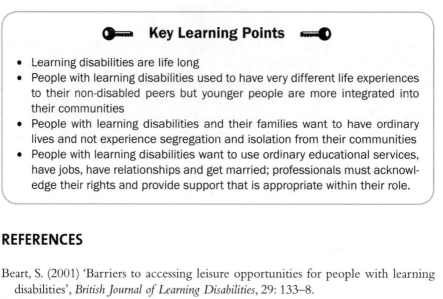

O━ Key Learning Points ━O

- Learning disabilities are life long
- People with learning disabilities used to have very different life experiences to their non-disabled peers but younger people are more integrated into their communities
- People with learning disabilities and their families want to have ordinary lives and not experience segregation and isolation from their communities
- People with learning disabilities want to use ordinary educational services, have jobs, have relationships and get married; professionals must acknowledge their rights and provide support that is appropriate within their role.

REFERENCES

Beart, S. (2001) 'Barriers to accessing leisure opportunities for people with learning disabilities', *British Journal of Learning Disabilities*, 29: 133–8.

Carers Act (1995) London: HMSO.

Carers and Disabled Children Act (2000) London: HMSO.

Carers UK (2010) *How do I get Help?: Your Guide to a Carers Assessment.* [online] Available from http://www.carersuk.org/Information/Helpwithcaring/Carersassessmentguide, accessed 03.04.2011.

Childcare Act (2006) London: HMSO.

Clarke, J., Seamer, J., Jones, D. and Scarborough, K. (2007) 'Trusting people: families leading services', *PMLD Link*, 19 (1): 7–10.

Cook, T., Swain, J. and French, S. (2001) 'Voices from segregated schooling: towards an inclusive education system', *Disability and Society*, 16 (2): 293–310.

Department for Children, Schools and Families (DCSF) (2003) *Every Child Matters.* London: Department for Children, Schools and Families.

Department for Children, Schools and Families (DCSF) (2006) *Duty to Provide Information, Advice and Assistance: Guidance for Local Authorities Childcare Act 2006.* London: Department for Children, Schools and Families.

Department for Children, Schools and Families (DCSF) (2008) *Bullying Involving Children with Special Educational Needs and Disabilities Safe to Learn: Embedding Anti-bullying Work in Schools*, London: Department for Children, Schools and Families.

Department for Work and Pensions (2010) 'Work choice programme'. [online] Available from http://www.direct.gov.uk/en/DisabledPeople/Employmentsupport/WorkSchemesAndProgrammes/DG_4001973, accessed 20.03.2011.

Department of Health (2001) *Valuing People: A New Strategy for Learning Disability for the 21st Century.* London: Department of Health.

Department of Health (2007a) *Putting People First: A Shared Vision and Commitment to the Transformation of Adult Social Care*. [online] Available from http://www.dh.gov.uk/en/Publicationsandstatistics/Publications/PublicationsPolicyAndguidance/DH_081118, Accessed 21.01.2010.

Department of Health (2007b) *Key Information for Professionals about the Transitions Processes for Disabled Young People*. [online] Available from http://www.transitioninfonetwork.org.uk/PDF/Transition_Guide_For_All_Services.pdf, accessed 20.03.2011.

Department of Health (2008) *Carers at the Heart of the 21st Century Families and Communities: A Caring System On Your Side, A Life of Your Own*. London: Department of Health.

Department of Health (2009a) *Valuing People Now – a New Three Year Strategy for People with Learning Disabilities*. London: Department of Health.

Department of Health (2009b) *Valuing Employment Now: Real Jobs for People with Learning Disabilities*. [online] Available from http://www.dh.gov.uk/en/Publicationsandstatistics/Publications/PublicationsPolicyAndGuidance/DH_101401, accessed 21.07.2010.

Department of Health and Department for Education and Skills (2007) *Good Practice Guidance on Working with Parents with a Learning Disability*. [online] Available from http://www.dh.gov.uk/en/Publicationsandstatistics/Publications/PublicationsPolicyAndGuidance/DH_075119, accessed 21.07.2010.

Directgov (2011) *Sure Start Children's Centres*. [online] Available from http://www.direct.gov.uk/en/Parents/Preschooldevelopmentandlearning/NurseriesPlaygroupsReceptionClasses/DG_173054, accessed 19.03.2011.

Emerson, E., Malam S., Davies, I. and Spencer, K. (2005) *Adults with Learning Difficulties in England 2003/4*. [online] Available at http://www.ic.nhs.uk/statistics-and-data-collections/social-care/adult-social-care-information/adults-with-learning-difficulties-in-england-2003-2004, accessed 03.04.2011.

Foster, C. (2009) 'Employing people with learning disabilities', *Equal Opportunities Review*, 190. [online] Available from http://www.eortrial.co.uk/default.aspx?id=1116246, accessed 20.08.2010.

Foundation for People with Learning Disabilities (2006) *This is What We Want*. [online] Available from http://www.learningdisabilities.org.uk/publications/?esctl544701_entryid5=15053&char=T accessed, 15.03.2010.

Gloucestershire Multi Agency Transition Group (2011) *The Gloucestershire Multi Agency Transition Pathway*. [online] Available from http://www.gloucestershire.gov.uk/index.cfm?articleid=13166, accessed 07.04.2011.

HM Government and Department of Health (2010) *Real Lives, Real Talent, Real Jobs*. [online] Available from http://www.valuingpeoplenow.dh.gov.uk/content/getting-a-job/employability-hub/good-case-studies, accessed 22.10.2010.

Highland Council (2008) *My Transition Guide for Parents, Professionals and Partnership Services*. [online] Available from http://www.highland.gov.uk/NR/rdonlyres/C4A1C8E0-577A-431E-8C63-500DFDC4BF32/0/transitionguideppp.pdf, accessed 20.03.2011.

Hollins, S., Attard, M.T., Von Fraunhofer, N., McGuigan, S. and Sedgwick, P. (1998) 'Mortality in people with learning disability: risks, causes and death certification findings in London', *Developmental Medicine and Child Neurology*, 40 (1): 50–6.

McCausland, D., Guerin, S., Dodd, P., Donohoe, C., Garvey, R., O'Donoghue, I. and Tyrrell, J. (2008) 'An assessment of the specialised health, social care and support needs of older people with intellectual disabilities', Paper presentation IASSID Congress Cape Town. Abstract, *Journal of Intellectual Disability Research,* 52 (8/9): 648.

Mencap (2001) *No Ordinary Life.* London: Mencap.

Mencap (2006) *Breaking Point: Families Still Need a Break.* London: Mencap.

Mencap (2007) *Bullying Wrecks Lives: the experiences of children and young people with learning disabilities.* London: Mencap.

Mencap (2009) *It's Good to Live Somewhere you feel Safe and Happy.* [online] Available from http://www.mencap.org.uk/landing.asp?id=40&type=text, accessed 01.01.2010.

Mencap (n.d.) *Experience of Diagnosis.* [online] Available from http://www.mencap.org.uk/page.asp?id=58, accessed 18.03.2011.

Michael, J. (2008) *Healthcare for All: Independent Inquiry into Access to Healthcare for People with Learning Disabilities.* [online] Available from http://www.iahpld.org.uk/, accessed 12.19.2010.

O'Bryan, A. and Beyer, S. (2005) *Valued in Public. Helping People with Learning Disabilities to Work in Public Bodies.* London: Mencap.

Office of National Statistics (2011) *Unemployment.* [online] Available from http://www.statistics.gov.uk/cci/nugget.asp?id=12, accessed 20.03.2011.

Robertson, J., Emerson, E., Hatton, C., Elliott, J., McIntosh, B., Swift, P., Krijnen-Kemp, E., Towers, C., Romeo, R., Knapp, M., Sanderson, H., Routledge, M., Oakes, P. and Joyce, T. (2005) *The Impact of Person Centred Planning.* Lancaster: Institute for Health Research, Lancaster University.

Scarborough, K. (2005) 'Complex People, Complex Risk', MSc Dissertation: University of Manchester.

Scope (2007) *An Introduction to Ageing and Cerebral Palsy.* Milton Keynes: SCOPE.

Special Educational Needs and Disability Act (2001). London: HMSO.

Stars in the Sky (2005) *Stars in the Sky.* [online] Available from http://www.starsinthesky.co.uk/, accessed 15.03.2010.

Strydom, A. and Hassiotis, A. (2003) 'Diagnostic instruments for dementia in older people with intellectual disability in clinical practice', *Ageing and Mental Health,* 7(6): 431–7.

Valuing People Support Team (2004) *Day Services Modernisation Toolkit Part One.* [online] Available from http://www.library.nhs.uk/learningdisabilities/ViewResource.aspx?resID=29707&tabID=288&catID=1122, accessed 15.03.2010.

Wilkinson, H., Kerr, D., Cunningham, C. and Rae, C. (2004) *Support for People with Learning Difficulties in Residential Settings who Develop Dementia.* York: Joseph Rowntree Foundation.

Working Together with Parents Network and Norah Fry (2009) *Supporting Parents with Learning Disabilities and Learning Difficulties Stories of Positive Practice.* Bristol: Norah Fry Research Centre.

5 ENABLING FAMILIES: A MODEL OF HELPING

Neil Summers

INTRODUCTION

As discussed in earlier chapters, policy and principles concerning the support for parents of children with learning disabilities has changed over the past decade. Parents have been at the forefront of these developments advocating for and on behalf of their children and challenging public services to provide adequate and effective resources. There have also been changes in some of the concepts and models used to develop services, with the emergence of person centred approaches and, more recently, individualised budgets. However, the influence of these changes is difficult to substantiate. For instance, Finch and Groves (1983) suggested that the care of children with disabilities in the UK almost always means care by another family member, and this family member is nearly always a woman. Have circumstances changed for families supporting children with learning disabilities? The way in which many services in the UK operate necessitates a referral from a GP or other professional. Parents with children with learning disabilities are forced in many situations to let professionals into their lives in order to gain access to a range of services. The consequence of this is the realisation that their needs are different from other families and their children may need specialist support.

The constant need to build new relationships with different workers has been a feature of service provision for many years (Dale, 1996). This chapter will focus on the effective help for parents with children with learning disabilities.

FAMILIES AND CHILDREN WITH LEARNING DISABILITIES

Chapters 2 and 4 discussed how some interventions have changed, aiming to build and sustain collaborative relationships with families. Alongside these changes, there has been a shift in the way that some families are depicted in the literature. The main thrust of these changes relates to a shift from a pathological, atypical parental reaction to a typical, common parental reaction. The pathological view suggests that parents react atypically to a child with a disability. Well-reported reactions of parents include denial, anger, sorrow, and over-protection. Gartner, Lipsky and Turnbull (1991) reported that professionals suggest that parents overprotect the child and often seek in-depth information on their child's disability and will 'shop around' for a second opinion. It is claimed that parents deny the reality of the situation and grieve for the loss of the idealised child. Parents who appear to be coping well with the situation are said to be overcompensating to reduce their sense of guilt. Daniels-Mohring and Lambie (1993) suggest that the anger that some parents present masks the guilt and sorrow they feel as a result of their child's disability. These claims by researchers are so prevalent that it would appear that all parents experience this range of experiences. Little attention is paid to the influence of economic or cultural circumstances and their impact on the family. Research in the 1980s began to challenge the negative view that was a prevalent feature of the research at that time. Furthermore, Sabbeth and Leventhal (1984) found that research focussed on parental reactions to disability rarely included control groups of families that did not have a disability. This prevents any meaningful comparison to other families' reactions to children. Vance et al. (1980) suggest that when control groups are used in research related to families' experiences of children with disability, the results do not demonstrate marked differences in functioning between families with and without children with disabilities.

It has been suggested that the presence of a child with learning disabilities may affect family dynamics (Trivette et al., 1990). McCallion and Toseland (1993) suggest that specific 'stressors' affect families with children with learning disabilities. Intagliata and Doyle (1984) argue that these 'stressors' are not experienced by other families. They are claimed to be caused by emotional strain, marital discord, sibling conflict, difficult developmental transitions, unresponsive service delivery systems and permanency-planning concerns (McCallion and Toseland, 1993). However, the concept of stress is not defined, even though it has become a common term (McConkey et al., 2008). Parents with children with learning disabilities are thought to experience greater stress reactions than other parents (Byrne and Cunningham, 1985). There are few explanations, however, regarding the variations in these reactions, as Grant et al. noted: 'despite the sophistication and considerable explanatory power of some models of stress process, there has been a tendency within the research community to view caring in pathological terms' (1998: 59). Attempts have been made to explore these experiences in more depth by describing parents' experiences and relating them to stages, similar to grief and mourning (see, for example, Parkes and Weiss, 1983). These general descriptors have been related to the many reactions parents of children with learning disabilities experience. It is thought that these experiences are reactions to the loss of their 'expected' child. These expectations are generally linked to the expected gender and ability of the child, and parents may be disappointed because their child does not look like the stereotypical 'perfect blue eyed boy' (Pushcel, 1991).

However, these experiences do not always equate to negative feelings towards their children. It is not uncommon, for example, for parents to resent the impairment, but continue to express feelings of love for their child (Cunningham and Davis, 1985). Davis et al. (1989) focussed on mothers' constructions of their children, and highlighted that parental awareness that their child with impairment is different from others need not imply negativity from the parents. Bruce et al. (1994) compared the experiences of three cohorts of parents. Their findings suggested that the grieving process should be considered as a continuous aspect of parents' experiences. Additionally, they found that the types of reaction varied considerably among the cohorts: 'there is joy and pride in the child's special progress, but for some the continuous strain is almost overwhelming' (Bruce et al., 1994: 49).

Some of the literature depicts negative parental reactions to the birth of a child with learning disabilities (Olshansky, 1962; Beck et al., 2004). These studies report a number of negative feelings – for example, sorrow, guilt and anger – related to the suggested 'shock' associated with the birth or diagnosis of a child. However, there are also studies which discuss different perspectives (Scorgie and Sobsey, 2000; Hastings and Taunt, 2002). Hastings and Taunt (2002) suggest that positive parental outcomes, like personal growth, and negative outcomes, like parental stress, are independent of each other. Parents reported positive perceptions of their children while recognising the difficulties they were experiencing.

Quine and Pahl (1991) investigated the effect of specific impairments as causes of stress to families. Their findings suggested that high levels of stress correlated with multiple impairments and behaviour problems. Stress in parents related to variables that focussed on the child and the social and economic circumstances of the family. The most stressful factors affecting the children were behaviour problems, night-time disturbance, multiple impairments and the child having an unusual appearance. Economic circumstances of the family included social isolation, adversity, and worries over money. These reactions are mixed with other factors adding to parents' concerns. Parents are also concerned about the availability of services when they could no longer support their child.

Best Practice – Helping and Helping Relationships

One concept held by many as having the potential to change the way services are modelled is the notion of empowerment. Empowerment is a concept that has been embraced by many organisations that work with families. The concept of empowerment offers frameworks for the exploration and development of new methods, strategies and practices which contribute to families defining and solving their own problems. However, empowerment still seems to be problematic. It would appear to have widespread appeal, but empirical evidence is lacking as to how it can effect sustained change in social situations. It appears that one of the key elements of the empowerment process is strengthening and supporting families. One model closely aligned with empowerment is the 'Enabling Practice' model developed by Dunst et al. (1988). The foundation of this model focusses on and explores the different styles that may be utilised by family workers when supporting families.

The notion of family-centred services has been current in the UK since the 1990s. Central to the complex nature of supporting families are the professionals who provide help. Families play a vital role in the support of their children and adult family members with learning disabilities. Many families cope independently and require no formal support from family services, but some request and require various types of support. However, the debilitating effect of certain types of help, and the manner in which it is provided, has been well documented (Dale, 1996). Madden (1995), for example, suggests that many professionals are prejudiced, ambivalent and ignorant of the concerns, insights and strengths of parents. This often results in conflict and a breakdown of the relationship between families and providers (Fisher et al., 1983).

The need to alleviate these tensions and harmonise relationships has led many parents/professionals to advocate the use of broad-based family systems that focus on enabling families to build strengths and develop partnerships with workers who offer support (Dunst et al., 1988; Dunst et al., 1989; Case, 2001). The aim of support services should be to strengthen families' ability to cope effectively with life events (Dunst et al., 1994), enabling families to remain in control of their lives and become more self-reliant and less dependent on family workers and services.

Many family support systems purport to associate their service practices with effective helping strategies. However, analysis would suggest that many are paradoxical in nature. The stated philosophies and aims of these agencies contrast significantly with the experiences reported by parents (Fiske, 1993; Cunningham et al., 1999). It would appear that there is little evidence to support the claims made by many agencies currently offering support. Additionally, the extent to which parents understand family support systems has not been represented in the literature. The introduction of the Carers and Disabled Children Act 2000 and *Valuing People* (DoH 2001; 2009) will support the development of best practice and encourage the review of current support services for families.

WHEN PARENTS MAKE CONTACT WITH PROFESSIONALS

The study by Redmond et al. (2002) suggested that help can lead to parents feeling that they should be grateful for the support they are offered. Moreover, they suggest the parent is likely to feel indebted to the worker if they have to ask for rather than being offered help. It could be assumed that if parents paid for the service/help then they might react differently when asking for help. These debilitating effects can be reversed by what Dunst et al. (2008) refer to as a process of creating opportunities for competencies to be acquired as part of meeting needs, solving problems, or achieving aspirations. The promotion and enhancement of competencies that permit an individual or group to become better able to solve problems, meet needs, and achieve aspirations would be a crucial part of the support offered to parents at this stage of the helping process.

Parents' reactions to the discovery that their child has learning disabilities are discussed earlier in this chapter. These views as to the likely impact of a child with learning disabilities on the family may explain why some of the interviewees in a study by Summers (2009) experienced emotional issues when deciding they needed support. It could be argued that by asking for help you expose yourself and your family to the judgement of professionals. Summers (2009) claimed that the difficulties that parents experienced in supporting their children confirmed their thoughts about their child's needs. None of the parents in this study had been given a formal diagnosis for their child before they decided they needed support (Summers, 2009). The turning point for these families appeared to be the realisation that they were unable to cope with their current situation, typically represented by the physical and/or emotional issues of supporting their child having an effect on their individual situations. Although it is recognised that families' experiences cannot and never will be typical, the difference in Summers' study (2009) was that their children were developing alongside their peers. This often resulted in parents in this study asking or being asked questions (by family, friends or workers) about their child's development. Moreover, parents of children without learning disabilities would be exposed to these experiences but would not have to deal with any of the issues related to their child's delayed development. As well as coming to terms with the possibility that they needed help, the parents in this study also dealt with the realisation that the help required was related to their child's developmental delay. Given that these experiences could be challenging for parents, a number of them found it difficult continually to relate their story about their child to numerous workers. It is clear to see that these children did not just suddenly acquire learning disabilities. The identification of learning disabilities is a progressive cultural practice, it is the socio-economic conditions and 'disablism' that contribute to the exclusion that the child and their parents experience. As it is difficult to make any firm conclusions about how parents react to the birth of a child with a disability, or news that their child has learning disabilities, it would appear appropriate to offer choices related to support at this stage. The important lesson to learn with regard to the helping process is that there is not a standard family and that each family experiences events and reacts to this news according to their values, culture, beliefs and resources. It is also important for services to be responsive to family requests for help to enable parents to begin to build early relationships with workers that promote the acquisition of effective behaviours that decrease the need for help, thus making the family more competent and more capable (Dempsey and Dunst, 2004).

SECURING HELP

Following the decision that they required help, many parents find it difficult to make contact with services. When help is established it is difficult to ascertain the effects on the parents of continually having to tell their story to different workers (Summers 2010). There is little written about the effect of parents being continually asked to explore their child's developmental history. However, parents are likely to tell different stories to different people because they do not have one story to tell. A parent may for example tell one story to a portage worker (pre-school home teachers) and a different one to a social worker. Parents appear to be saying that they find it intrusive and difficult to convey personal information to so many different workers offering help, as they find it difficult to build relationships with so many different professionals.

Making the decision to seek professional help is one of the many transitions parents face as their children grow. These transitions include the birth of a child, the news that the child has a learning disability, working through the emotions related to a diagnosis, establishing the need for help, and supporting the child into education. Each transition gives rise to various support requirements and to meet these parents may need to access formal and informal networks. Moving into these networks will again mean sharing intimate details about their family with many different people. This appears to be the area that has the potential to cause emotional trauma and conflict for the interviewees in Summers' 2010 study. If these events are matched by negative perceptions about the availability of appropriate support, these negative emotions could be unresolved (Redmond et al., 2002; Summers, 2010) and are entangled with the realisation that by asking for help parents are revealing themselves and their feelings to the outside world. A possible way of alleviating these concerns would be to:

- help families write a FAQ sheet about themselves to send to professional prior to a first meeting
- ensure that the helper reads previous records or discusses this information with previous helpers
- prevent repetitive information gathering by writing to parents before a visit suggesting information that they may need to know about families
- ensure that this information is passed on to other workers (sometimes known as a handover)
- ensure it is understood that a local, consistent and organised network of formal and informal services is needed to support the individual needs of families moving through these transitions.

The need to build a consistent relationship with a worker appears important to parents. Summers (2010) found that carers were not offered any choices in relation to professional type, gender, age or expertise of workers. Summers (2009) identified evidence of strengthening bonds in families, despite the often stressful emotional experience. Carers described a deeper love and devotion to their children during this time. Parents also reported that despite increased levels of physical demands (because of caring for their child) they perceived changes associated with personal growth and maturity resulting from their experiences. These findings contribute to the body of evidence that supports the view that care giving can be satisfying and rewarding (Hastings and Taunt, 2002). One of the factors that may have influenced carers' experiences was the relationship some had developed with a particular worker. Summers (2009) identified that parents found the emotional support offered by workers at the time when they were experiencing reactions to the needs of their children as beneficial in helping them remain positive about their children.

Much has been written about the perceived shift in worker approaches associated with different models of service delivery (Barnes and Oliver, 1995; Case, 2001; Dunst et al., 2002). This shift is typified by a move away from the medical model towards different theoretical and conceptual models that underpin the way workers approach the support of families. In Summers' (2009) study parents talked in more general terms about what it felt like to be helped, and what the helper was like and the impressions they made. The ease with which parents were able to build relationships with workers appeared to be an important aspect of the relationship dynamic, (Summers, 2009). The strong personal characteristics of the workers – for example caring, comfortable, and easy to get to know – were thought to be key to a successful carer–worker relationship. These general impressions are significant since they felt it was important that workers were able to use these positive characteristics when building relationships with families. However, these general impressions are difficult to quantify and generalise. How, for example, can workers ensure that they are easy to get to know and are comfortable to be with? These attributes are not specifically linked to a particular, conscious approach adopted by a worker but appear to be personal traits that are considered helpful by parents when building relationships. It is interesting to note that some carers identified negative personal characteristics that weakened or resulted in a breakdown in relations with workers. Workers who were unfriendly or difficult to get to know, who appeared uninterested in families or were uncomfortable to be with manifested attributes that interviewees felt weakened and damaged their relations with them. It could be argued that workers who did not build strong relationships were not able to connect on a personal level with parents. Parents did not identify specific approaches that influenced the relationship but more subjective personal characteristics. Carers found it difficult to build new relationships when long-term workers were replaced or left the service.

Reflection Point 13

Parents suggested in the Summers study (2009) that they want staff who are caring and easy to get to know. However, these characteristics are not always easy to quantify.

Thinking about yourself, how would your behaviours and ways of working show that you are 'caring'? What would you do to ensure you are 'easy to get to know', have 'good communication skills', and 'gave accessible information'?

How would you terminate a long-term professional relationship to best support the next professional in developing an effective relationship?

You may have suggested that when people seeking help have strong emotional links with the person providing help these relationships are more likely to be successful. Summers' findings (2009) pose potentially difficult scenarios for services that employ workers to support parents. It is difficult to embed personal attributes into job roles and equally difficult to employ workers who have, or have the potential to develop, such characteristics. Conversely, carers reported dissatisfaction with the workers perceived as judgemental, inadequate listeners and poor at communicating ideas to families. Some parents felt that their parenting style was being challenged when workers advised them how to manage their child's behaviour. This is a common experience of parents, and workers need to be tactful and diplomatic in the way they communicate their advice and recommendations about managing aspects of their children's behaviour with parents.

When workers adopt approaches that present themselves as experts, parental involvement can be limited. The worker as an expert can take control of the relationship using their perceived expertise to control and take responsibility away from the carer. Although taking control away from parents can be useful when parents want/need expert opinions (this may be as a result of emotional confusion), this approach can result in a conflicting worker/carer goals for the child (Case, 2001).

Reflection Point 14

Reflect on some of the unhelpful strategies explored in the previous paragraph. For example, thinking about yourself, what biases influence your own relationships with parents? What negative ideas do you hold about parents of children with learning disabilities?

Practical skills of workers are valued by many parents and this was a highlight of the findings in Summers' study (2009). Activities related to respite provision – for example play schemes and respite holidays, swimming sessions and other social events – are very important to parents but are often riddled with administration requirements, like liability insurance and volunteer training. One of the knock-on effects of workers taking responsibility for the children on outings and play schemes appeared to be a stronger working relationship with families. Relationships with children and families can be strengthened because the worker gets to know the child better on such activities. This corresponds with evidence of the importance of workers getting to know children, from other parents who have reported dissatis-faction with this aspect of their relationship with workers (Case, 2001). The parents' perception that a worker wants to, can and ought to build a closer relationship with the child appears to be an important feature of supporting families. It could be argued that parents who perceive strong relationships between the child and a worker can contribute to them feeling that workers are part of their struggle.

However, Dowling and Dolan (2001) reported that one carer suggested that their worker was easy to get to know and friendly but did not meet the perceived needs of the family. It is difficult to measure how much these factors influence the parent/worker relationship but they appeared to be highly valued by almost all families. What does emerge from the literature is a link between a strong worker/parent relationship and workers who clearly stated what they could and could not do with and for families. Additionally, workers who are realistic and honest with parents about resources and aspects of their child's development were likewise valued in some of the literature (see Dowling and Dolan, 2001; Dempsey and Dunst, 2009; Summers, 2009). However, what is unclear in the literature are the factors that cause conflict in worker/parents relationships. Parents report general factors and are not specific about the causal factors related to conflict. It was not clear, for example, whether areas of conflict are specially associated with a worker's approach or the characteristics of that approach. If, for example, a worker was utilising an expert model (Case, 2001) that is criticised for taking away the control from parents, but that worker was viewed as open and honest, would these attributes counter the areas of conflict? Additionally, working in the best interest of the parent may not always address the child's needs.

Moreover, parents appear to value the personal characteristics of workers more than any particular approach (Summers, 2009). They value the softer aspects of relationships often associated with personal rather than professional contacts. Although Summers' findings (2009) are difficult to generalise it could be suggested that it is essential that workers have or develop personal characteristics which will help them to build and sustain relationships with families. Additionally, it could also be suggested that workers in this study were skilled and were utilising both a professional approach and personal characteristics that strengthened worker/carer relationships. I can identify situations as a practitioner when it was more important for me to befriend families rather than simply to be a professional. If workers, for some families, are their only contacts to discuss family issues, it may be important for workers to step outside of the professional boundaries that shape worker approaches.

THE EDUCATION OF PARENTS

Linked to the help received and resources for carers is the need to offer education to parents with children with learning disabilities. Summers (2009) found that parents wanted to maintain and develop new skills that would help with the care of their children. It is apparent from the earlier discussion that parents sought information from workers about their child's needs in and around the time they were given a clear indication that their child had a disability. Parents want to continue to develop their knowledge base and used various avenues in these pursuits. Read (2002) indicated that parents with children with disabilities developed expert knowledge, skills and perceptions about their children's needs. However, the availability of resources to support this group of parents is limited. Funding for training and education in health and social care is typically controlled by statutory services (Mallett, 2006). Carers often rely on informal networks to develop and share knowledge and skills. Access to formal education has been problematic for parents, and people and adults with learning disabilities (Summers et al., 2004). One initiative that has attempted to develop and support parents and adults in higher education is based at the University of the West England, Bristol. Funding for a work-based certificate programme was secured from the local Workforce Development Confederation for parents and adults with learning disabilities. The benefits of this initiative suggested that there were opportunities for reciprocal learning in the groups (Scarborough et al., 2006). Parents who studied on the programme are now actively involved in curricula and write and present at national conferences (Summers et al., 2004). However, the continued funding for these modules has not been secured.

A MODEL OF HELPING

This chapter has illuminated the complex nature of asking for, receiving and building helping relationships for parents with children with learning disabilities. The key feature of this process appears to be the partnership between the family and worker. The elements that feature in the development of effective partnerships are identified in Figure 5.1.

Figure 5.2 clearly identifies the key elements related to disempowering experiences of parents and relates to indicators that many helping acts can result in negative outcomes for families (Summers, 2009). Moreover, families reported that when workers took control of their lives this affected their self-esteem, with workers conveying a sense that the family was inferior, incompetent and inadequate (Dunst et al., 1989). The process related to the

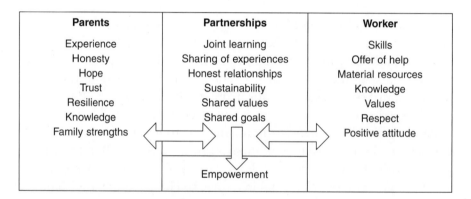

FIGURE 5.1   *Elements of Empowerment: Parent*

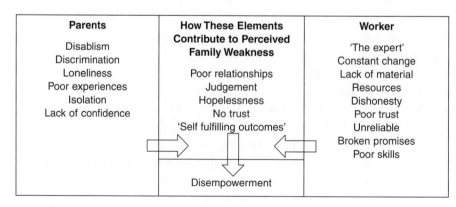

FIGURE 5.2   *Elements of Disempowerment: Parent and Workers*

empowerment of families has been developed by Summers (2009) into a model of helping (see Figure 5.3).

This model (Figure 5.3) indicates that the empowerment of families with children with learning disabilities is part of a process which involves the resources that families/workers and society offer to develop and sustain partnerships. These resources help families to take control and be in a position to act on matters that affect their lives. The combination of the resources that are available and accessible to families will help to build partnerships. This partnership is a symbiotic relationship in which the skilled worker derives satisfaction from doing their job well and is appreciated by the families, while the family is sustained and empowered and made strong by the partnership. Resources are a joint capital of the family–professional partnership. Resources include the human resources offered by workers, matched with material resources that can be used to support

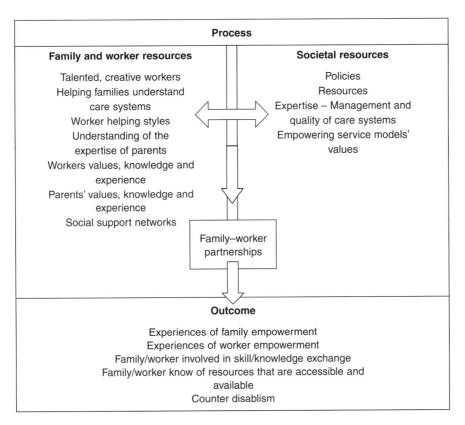

FIGURE 5.3   *A Model of Helping*

families. It is also important to note that effective helping for parents may not always meet the child's needs as their needs can be different and children may be at risk if workers focus only on parents' perceptions.

The skills of the worker in this partnership are important. Parents appear to be asking for a worker who offers emotional rather than instrumental support (Kawachi et al., 2007). One feature of this model suggests that the socially skilled, emotionally intelligent worker was preferred to the technically skilled and experienced supporter. Thus, the helper's personal skill is in effect a resource to the family.

Reflection Point 15

Parents and children need workers with skills and knowledge but also emotional intelligence (EI). Many professionals would not have explored EI in their training. Do you know what EI means? Do you have a high level of EI? How do you know about your EI? If you are tempted to skip this reflective point maybe you are not as comfortable with the concepts of emotional intelligence as you could be. Wikipedia has a short but informative and critical section on emotional intelligence that is worth reading to start exploring what EI is.

We can, following the model of Figure 5.3, speak of relational resources (workers) and of societal resources, for example policies related to direct payments to parents with disabled children. In effect, access to what is available depends on the skill, knowledge and human qualities of the worker and the relationships that are enjoyed by both parties. There are two types of resources:

1   qualities, skills and approaches (we might see these as 'human practices')
2   materials/economic assets which are made accessible to the families by society.

In relation to qualities, skills and approaches, it is clear that educators and service providers need to prepare workers to build and sustain partnerships with families. However, some of these qualities are difficult to teach. Alongside the investment and development of human resources, it is important to develop and support the concept and principles of empowerment within organisations. There is little point in developing a skilled workforce unless these workers are supported at an operational and structural level (Michael Report, 2008).

The successful deployment of family and worker resources matched by material and economic assets will help to build effective partnerships. The outcomes in this model (Figure 5.3) are that the child and the family are immunised from some of the toxic effects of direct and indirect discrimination; the family's knowledge, skills, experiences and expertise are valued; and the worker increases their competencies. The model developed provides clear values for families, workers and services that will guide processes so that the outcome is the empowerment of families, empowered professionals, inclusion and joy for the disabled child, and an empowered community for all of us to live in.

CONCLUSION

The empowerment of families with children with learning disabilities is part of a process which involves the resources that families, workers and society offer to develop and sustain partnerships and inclusion. Resources include the human resources offered by workers (including practical skills) matched with material resources that can be used to support families. To enable this to happen partnerships are needed where professional power is understood. Partnerships are a symbiotic relationship and it is important that skilled workers derive satisfaction from doing their job well and the family is sustained, empowered and made strong by that partnership. To enable this to occur parents appear to be asking for a worker who offers emotional rather than instrumental support and it is the socially skilled and emotionally intelligent worker who was preferred to the technically skilled and experienced supporter. It is important to develop models which embrace principles of empowerment at individual and organisational levels to ensure that children and their families are immunised from some of the toxic effects of direct and indirect discrimination. Within this model the family's knowledge, skills, experiences and expertise must be valued. This increases the worker's competencies in working in enabling ways with families.

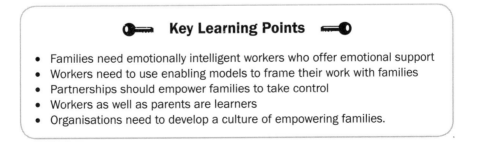

Key Learning Points

- Families need emotionally intelligent workers who offer emotional support
- Workers need to use enabling models to frame their work with families
- Partnerships should empower families to take control
- Workers as well as parents are learners
- Organisations need to develop a culture of empowering families.

REFERENCES

Barnes, C. and Oliver, M. (1995) 'Disability rights: rhetoric and reality in the UK', *Disability and Society*, 10 (1): 111–116.

Beck, A., Daley, D., Hastings, R. and Stevenson, J. (2004) 'Mothers' expressed emotion towards children with and without intellectual disabilities', *Journal of Intellectual Disability Research*, 48 (7): 628–38.

Bruce, E., Schultz, C., Smyrios, K. and Schultz, N. (1994) 'Grieving related to development: A preliminary comparison of three age cohorts of parents of children with intellectual disability', *British Journal of Medical Psychology*, 67: 37–52.

Byrne, E.A. and Cunningham, C.C. (1985) 'The effects of mentally handicapped children on families – a conceptual review', *Journal of Child Psychology and Psychiatry*, 26 (6): 847–64.

Case, S. (2001) 'Learning to partner, disabling conflict: early indications of an improving relationship between parents and professionals with regard to service provision for children with learning disabilities', *Disability, Handicap and Society*, 16 (6): 837–54.

Cunningham, C. and Davis, H. (1985) *Working with Parents: Frameworks for Collaboration*. Milton Keynes: Open University Press.

Cunningham, P.B., Henggeler, S.W., Brondino, M.J. and Pickrel, S.G. (1999) 'Testing underlying assumptions of the family empowerment perspective', *Journal of Child and Family Studies*, 8 (4): 437–49.

Dale, N. (1996) *Working with Families of Children with Special Needs: Partnership and Practice*. London: Routledge.

Daniels-Mohring, D. and Lambie, R. (1993) 'Dysfunctional families of the student with special needs', *Focus on Exceptional Children*, 25 (5.5): 1–11.

Davis, H., Stroud, A. and Green, L. (1989) 'Child characterisation sketch. International', *Journal of Personal Construct Psychology*, 2: 323–37.

Dempsey, I. and Dunst, C.J. (2004) 'Help giving styles and parent empowerment in families with a young child with a disability', *Journal of Intellectual and Development Disabilities*, 29:1 40–51.

Dempsey, I. and Dunst, C.J. (2005) 'Help giving styles and the parent empowerment in families with a young child with a disability', *The Journal of Intellectual and Developmental Disability*, 29 (1): 40–51.

Department of Health (2001) *Valuing People: A New Strategy for Learning Disability for the 21st Century*. London: Department of Health.

Department of Health (2009) *Valuing People Now: A New Three-year Strategy for People with Learning Disabilities*. London: Department of Health.

Dowling, M. and Dolan, L. (2001) 'Families with children with disabilities – inequalities and the social model' *Disability and society*, 16 (1): 21–35.

Dunst, C.J., Trivette, C.M. and Deal, A.G. (1988) *Enabling and Empowering Families: Principles and Guidelines for Practice*. Cambridge, MA: Brookline Books.

Dunst, C.J., Trivette, C.M., Gordon, N. and Plether, L.L. (1989) 'Building and Mobilizing Informal Support Networks', in G.H. Singer and L.K. Irvin (eds), *Support for Caregiving Families: Enabling Positive Adaptation to Disability*. Baltimore: Paul H Brookes Publishing.

Dunst, C.J., Trivette, C.M. and Deal, A.G. (1994) 'Resource-based family-centered intervention practices', in C.J. Dunst, C.M. Trivette and A.G. Deal (eds), *Supporting and Strengthening Families: Methods, Strategies and Practices*. Cambridge, MA: Brookline Books.

Dunst, C.J., Boyd, K., Trivette, C.M. and Hamby, D.W. (2002) 'Family-oriented program models and professional helpgiving practices', *Family Relations*, 51, 221–9.

Dunst, C.J., Trivette, C.M., and Hamby, D.W. (2008) *Research Synthesis and Meta-analysis of Studies of Family-centered Practices* (Winterberry Monograph Series). Asheville, NC: Winterberry Press.

Finch, J. and Groves, D. (1983) *A Labour of Love: Women, Work, and Caring*. London: Routledge and Kegan Paul.

Fisher, J.D., Nadler, A. and DePaulo, B.M. (1983) *New Directions in Helping*. New York: Academic Press.

Fiske, S. (1993) 'Controlling other people: the impact of power on stereotyping', *American Psychology*, 48 (6): 621–8.

Gartner, A., Lipsky, D.K. and Turnbull, A.P. (1991) *Supporting Families with a Child with Disabilities: An International Outlook*. New York: Brooks.

Grant, G., Ramcharan, P., McGrath, M., Nolan, M. and Keady, J. (1998) 'Rewards and gratifications among family caregivers: towards a refined model of caring and coping', *Journal of Intellectual Disability Research*, 42: 58–71.

Hastings, R.P. and Taunt, H.M. (2002) 'Positive perceptions in families of children with developmental disabilities', *American Journal on Mental Retardation*, 107 (2): 116–27.

Intagliata, J. and Doyle, N. (1984) 'Enhancing social support for parents of developmentally disabled children: training in interpersonal problem solving skills', *Mental Retardation*, 22 (1): 4–11.

Kawachi, I., Subramanian, S.V. and Kim, D. (2007) *Social Capital and Health*. London: SpringerLink.

Madden, P. (1995) 'Why parents: how parents', *British Journal of Learning Disabilities*, 23: 90–3.

Mallett, S. (2006) *Information Paper on NHS Funding of Workforce Development and its Implications for the Widening Participation in Learning Strategy*. London: Widening Participation in Learning Strategy Unit, DoH (WPSU17).

McCallion, P. and Toseland, R.W. (1993) 'Empowering families of adolescents and adults with developmental disabilities', *Families in Society: The Journal of Contemporary Human Services*, 37: 579–87.

McConkey, R., Truesdale-Kennedy, M., Chang, M., Jarrah, S. and Shukri, R. (2008) 'The impact on mothers of bringing up a child with intellectual disabilities: A cross-cultural study', *International Journal of Nursing Studies*, 45 (1): 65–74.

Michael Report (2008) *Healthcare for All: Report of the Independent Enquiry into Access to Healthcare for People with Learning Disabilities*. London: Department of Health.

Olshansky, J. (1962) 'Chronic sorrow: a response to having a mentally deficient child', *Social Casework*, 43: 190–3.

Parent and Disabled Child Act (2000) London: HMSO.

Parkes, C.M. and Weiss, R. (1983) *Recovery from Bereavement*. New York: Basic Books.

Pushcel, S. (1991) 'Ethical considerations relating to prenatal diagnosis of foetuses with Down's Syndrome', *Mental Retardation*, 29: 185–90.

Quine, L. and Pahl, J. (1991) 'Stress and coping in mothers caring for a child with severe learning difficulties: a test of Lazarus' transactional model of coping', *Journal of Community and Applied Social Psychology*, 1: 57–70.

Read, J. (2002) 'Will the carers and Disabled Children Act 2000 make a difference to the lives of disabled children and their carers?', *Child: Care, Health and Development*. 28 (4): 273–5.

Redmond, C., Spoth, R. and Trueau, L. (2002) 'Family and community-level predictors of parent support seeking', *Journal of Community Psychology*, 30 (2): 153–71.

Sabbeth, B.F. and Leventhal, J.M. (1984) 'Marital adjustment to chronic childhood illness: a critique of the literature', *Paediatrics*, 73 (6): 762–8.

Scarborough, K., Broussine, E. and Summers, N. (2006) 'Taking control: university education helps people with learning disabilities "make change happen"', *Learning Disability Practice*, 9 (9): 28–31.

Scorgie, K. and Sobsey, D. (2000) 'Transformational outcomes associated with parenting children who have disabilities', *Mental Retardation*, 38: 195–206.

Summers, N. (2009) 'Parental perceptions of enabling strategies of services supporting children with learning disabilities: an ethnographic study', unpublished Thesis, University of the West of England, Bristol.

Summers, N. (2010) 'The ethnography of help – supporting families with children with intellectual disabilities', 3rd IASSID Europe Conference Integrating Biomedical and Psycho Social Educational Perspectives , 20–22 October, 2010, Rome, Italy.

Summers, N., Smith, M., Hogarth, S. and Scarborough, K. (2004) 'User involvement in health and social care'. Paper presented at *User Involvement in Health and Social Care Practice, Education and Research*, 21 January, Middlesex University.

Trivette, C.M., Dunst, C.J., Deal, A.G., Wilson Hamer, A. and Propst, S. (1990) 'Assessing family strengths and family functioning style', *Topics in Early Childhood Special Education*, 10 (1): 16–35.

Vance, J.C., Fazan, L.E., Satterwhite, B. and Pless, I.B. (1980) 'Effects of nephritic syndrome on the family: a controlled study', *Paediatrics*, 64: 948–55.

6 BUILDING POSITIVE RELATIONSHIPS WITH PEOPLE WITH LEARNING DISABILITIES

Eric Broussine

INTRODUCTION

Engaging with people with learning disabilities at a personal yet professional level can be demanding but is ultimately rewarding for both parties. It is a human right for people to have a sense of belonging and to have lasting, genuine friendships, to feel valued, liked and respected. All too often people with learning disabilities miss out on opportunities to form lasting friendships and positive relationships, losing their basic human right to engage in and enjoy everything that friendship brings. This chapter explores the tensions between being person centred and according people with learning disabilities respect while maintaining professional boundaries around the 'friendship' aspect of the relationship. However, working at a task-orientated level in which there is a degree of emotional detachment that insidiously objectifies and dehumanises people in care is not regarded as helpful in promoting a therapeutic relationship. Developing positive relationships with an attitude of person centredness and humanistic principles which respects the 'personhood' of the individual not only brings rewards for people with learning disabilities and their carers but also promotes a culture of mutual respect and acceptance. Although healthcare staff will not and cannot be expected to form lasting friendships when people with learning disabilities are admitted into hospital, there is an expectation that practitioners will want to ensure that people's experiences of healthcare staff in hospital or other healthcare settings are positive, supportive and safe. The purpose of this chapter, therefore, is to raise awareness of the interpersonal and communication qualities and skills that professional carers need to develop and apply when people with learning disabilities access primary or secondary healthcare and social care settings.

This chapter is divided into four sections. The first section will explore three core attributes and qualities of the practitioner (after Rogers, 1957), namely congruence, unconditional positive regard (UPR) and empathic understanding. According to Rogers (1957) these conditions are regarded as necessary for promoting an effective therapeutic relationship. The second section will examine how these qualities can be applied by the practitioner through their verbal, para-verbal and non-verbal behaviour. Egan (2007) uses the term 'micro-skills' as a framework for learning individual components of listening and attending. The third section discusses the importance of self-awareness and the therapeutic use of self. It also outlines the importance of reflective practice and how being a reflective practitioner enhances best practice and the therapeutic environment. The fourth section elaborates upon the relationship between the above three sections and the promotion of self-esteem in people with learning disabilities.

THE THREE CORE CONDITIONS OF CONGRUENCE, UNCONDITIONAL POSITIVE REGARD AND EMPATHIC UNDERSTANDING

While it is recognised that health and social care practitioners are not 'therapists' and are not expected to enter into deep psychological, thera-peutic relationships, an awareness, working knowledge and application of Rogers' three core conditions (1957) should underpin best practice when forming positive working relationships with people with learning disabilities. The conditions offer a framework around the potential tensions between practitioners being 'friendly', person centred and approachable while maintaining professional boundaries and recognising their key responsibilities within the context of health and social care provision.

Rogers (1957) wrote a significant paper that conceptualised the conditions and attitudes necessary for an effective psychotherapeutic relationship. In effect, he clarified the ingredients of the therapeutic relationship and made the conditions accessible to others (Thorne, 1992, cited in Thomas and Woods, 2003). The three core conditions are congruence, unconditional positive regard (UPR) and empathic understanding. Each core condition will be defined, explored and evaluated in terms of caring for people with learning disabilities.

Congruence

Congruence can be defined as rapport within oneself, an internal and external consistency which is perceived by others as sincerity, genuineness, realness, transparency, authenticity and spontaneity. It means coming into a direct personal encounter with the person, meeting and interacting with them on a person-to-person basis. When we are congruent, we are demonstrating to other people as well as to ourselves that we are open and honest. We are being genuine, true to our feelings, thoughts and behaviours and not pretending or hiding behind a level of expertise, a personal facade or using our professionalism as an obstacle to forming a positive working relationship. A practitioner who is self-aware, reflective and intuitive will mean what they say and their feelings will match what is expressed. For example, a person with a learning disability may behave in a way that is perceived as offensive or hurtful to the practitioner. We are being congruent when we can express our feelings openly and honestly to the person and let them know how their behaviour makes us feel. If what we say verbally matches how we express it non-verbally, we are demonstrating congruence. Words, voice and body language give the same message. If the person with a learning disability experiences congruence from the practitioner, they in turn feel secure and safe to be themselves and a trusting, respectful relationship can develop.

Unconditional Positive Regard (UPR)

Often known as warm acceptance, unconditional positive regard is about developing a warm, encouraging, accepting atmosphere, regarding the person unconditionally, without judgement or values, and trying to be open to the experiences of the person in a manner that expresses praise and a positive attitude. Acceptance means being willing to allow the person to express him or herself freely and openly and to accept them as a unique individual. This condition means respect and thus promotes a climate of safety for the person. UPR means valuing the humanity of the client and is not deflected in that valuing by any particular client behaviours. Many people with learning disabilities have not experienced unconditional warm acceptance from practitioners or the general public, rather they have experienced unequal 'doing to' instead of 'being with' relationships (Kwaitek et al., 2005). Invariably, people with learning disabilities will experience conditional positive regard instead; for example, positive regard is conditional on them behaving in a way that parents, carers and significant others expect them to behave and think. The person is not accepted for who they are but on condition that they behave only in ways approved by others. A person who only experiences conditional positive regard will constantly seek approval from other people.

Empathic Understanding

In explaining empathic understanding, Rogers said it was to 'sense the client's private world as if it were your own, without losing the "as if" quality.' (1957: 96). Empathy can be described as a way of being, imaginatively entering into another person's experiences and attempting to see the world from their perspective. Although impossible to achieve fully, even if the practitioner can only guess what a person may be experiencing would be demonstrating empathic understanding. The practitioner then communicates their understanding back to the individual and that, to some degree, the person's experiences are being understood. Empathy means being sensitive to the feelings of the other person, temporarily living in the other person's life, without being judgemental or prejudicial. For example, a practitioner is being empathic when they observe that a person with a learning disability is anxious and scared of being in a strange, hospital environment. The practitioner listens and acknowledges their feelings and communicates that understanding back to the person in a manner that they can understand. The person feels understood, accepted and begins to trust the practitioner. Having someone else really understand how you feel can be nurturing and healing, as people with learning disabilities often feel very much alone in their differentness from other people. Empathy builds trust and is a key quality in building a positive helping working relationship. Making human contact through attending, observing and listening are the means to demonstrating empathic understanding and 'being with' as described by Kwaitek et al. (2005) earlier.

Reflection Point 1.6

Reflect on a situation when you demonstrated one of the three core conditions with a patient.

How did you demonstrate the condition?

How did the patient respond?

What were the outcomes, for you and for the patient?

THE MICRO-SKILLS OF ATTENDING AND LISTENING

This section examines how the practitioner can demonstrate the core conditions in their verbal, non-verbal and para-verbal behaviour and in their everyday interactions with people with learning disabilities. A framework is suggested for building attending and active listening skills and, thus, the means to express your value base and competence in communicating and promoting the well-being of people with learning disabilities.

Egan (2007) examined in detail communication skills and coined the word 'micro-skills', as a way that helpers can learn the components of attending and listening. He defined attending as a process of 'being' with people, at both a physical and a psychological level. Cumbie (2001) argues that being with, being authentic and genuine with clients relates to being focussed on the needs of the client and if the practitioner can 'give' of themselves and fully participate in the interaction, then they are being humanistic and holistic in their caring relationships.

A focus on attending reinforces person centred practice and helps orientate away from task-driven and mechanistic methods of working and relating. Attending to clients lets them know you are with them, prepares you to listen intently to their concerns and to pick up on any verbal and non-verbal cues. This is especially important when interacting with people with severe and profound learning disabilities as the practitioner may only have non-verbal cues to rely on as a means of understanding the client. Effective attending invites people to trust you, reinforces mutual understanding and, if relaxed, encourages people to be more willing to open up.

SOLER

Egan (2007) used the acronym SOLER as a starting point or first level of attending:

S – Face the client *squarely*. Turning your body towards the person indicates presence and a willingness to engage and be involved. If sitting squarely is interpreted as being threatening, sitting at an angled position may be better.

O – Adopt an *open* posture. Folded arms and legs can indicate a defensive and a less involved stance towards the person. An open posture may indicate an increased willingness to listen. The importance is having an awareness of your posture and whether it conveys openness and availability.

L – *Lean* towards the other person. This further indicates 'being with' and interested in the other person. Leaning back and away from the person can indicate disinterest, even boredom. Leaning too far forward can appear threatening and intimidating. The idea is to be flexible with how you use your upper body in interactions.

E – Maintain good *eye* contact. Try and develop steady eye contact which conveys a message of wanting to be with the person. It is appropriate to look away at times but be aware of how much eye contact you maintain. Too little eye contact could indicate a lack of enthusiasm or uneasiness in wanting to be with the person.

R – Try to be *relaxed* in your interactions. If you fidget or use distracting facial expressions this may be an indicator of your nervousness and discomfort in being with the person. If you convey a relaxed or natural state, the person will also feel relaxed and comfortable.

The SOLER acronym is a useful framework and facilitates the learning of the micro-skills. Chambers (2003) discusses Non-Verbal Communication (NVC) and its use with people with learning disabilities. Having an increased awareness of your own non-verbal behaviours in practitioner–patient interactions heightens your awareness of the patient's NVC. You are then more skilled in noticing and interpreting cues and other behaviours. If a non-verbal person with a learning disability likes being with you this may be indicated through their behaviour – smiling, maintaining eye contact, their para-verbal utterances and close proximity. If a client cries out, shouts or bites themselves, this may suggest that the individual is in pain or expressing some other form of discomfort. Through the process of attending, the practitioner demonstrates that they want to be with the person, can learn more about them, and is then in a stronger position to meet their needs. In effect, the practitioner learns the value and the importance of 'being' with the client at a physical as well as a psychological level.

If you combine active listening to your repertoire of attending skills then you are more likely to be successful in your engagement with people with learning disabilities. Active listening is vital to the development of effective communication (Burnard, 1997) and is active as opposed to passive because it involves conscious activities of the listener to try and understand the total message that is being sent. McNaughton et al. (2008) describe active listening as a multi-step process, involving the use of empathic comments, asking appropriate questions, and the use of paraphrasing and summarising that focusses on the client's story. Bryant (2009) reminds practice nurses of the importance of organising and promoting an environment that is conducive to listening by making time, minimising interruptions and engaging in a warm, quiet and private room. Other active listening skills are reflecting back key words and phrases, the feelings behind the words, and mirroring body language. Egan (2007) claims that there are four micro-skills of active listening:

- Observing and reading non-verbal behaviour, especially important when engaging with people with multiple and profound learning disabilities and limited verbal communication skills
- Listening and understanding clients' verbal messages
- Listening to the context, that is being aware of the social, cultural and environmental context of their life
- Listening to any contradictions and inconsistencies that may need to be challenged.

By providing a range of feedback methods we let the person know that we are listening attentively to their subjective experiences. This in turn builds trust and rapport in the relationship and assists in the healing process (Boudreau et al., 2009). This level of listening is often referred to as empathic listening and further demonstrates congruence and warm acceptance of the client.

One of the many challenges of practitioners being active listeners occurs with clients who have limited or no verbal speech patterns, have a sensory impairment, have a profound physical as well as a learning disability or have autism. The practitioner has to rely on augmentative and/or alternative communication methods (see Chapter 7), the person's non-verbal behaviour and on other professionals or carers for gathering information. An individual with autism may give limited or no eye contact, but this should not be misinterpreted as not being interested or aware of their surroundings; a physical impairment can result in idiosyncratic body language that can easily be misunderstood; and someone with a hearing or visual impairment will have problems attending appropriately. Many people with learning disabilities may exhibit some of these non-verbal behaviours and they can compromise understanding, leading to premature termination of a 'conversation' or contact, which in turn compromises the caring relationship.

People with learning disabilities frequently experience non-helpful attending and listening from practitioners. They are likely to experience negative and stereotyped attitudes towards them and professionals often have lower expectations of them, believing that they are more child-like, dependent and less able (Fitzsimmons and Barr, 1997). These attitudes will be reflected in how well they listen to clients. Any preconceived opinions or biases the practitioner has about people with learning disabilities will inevitably 'leak' out through their verbal and non-verbal behaviours. However, if your attitude is person centred and you endeavour to raise your awareness of Rogers's (1957) core conditions, and you begin to apply them through skilled attending and active listening, you will be making an effort to promote the personhood of the individual with a learning disability. If you attend and actively listen you are engaging at a far deeper, emotional level with the client and are, according to Cumbie (2001), practicing the art of transpersonal caring, whereby the practitioner participates fully, recognising the value of using themself therapeutically in the caring–healing relationship. In concluding this section, it would seem that attending and active listening have far-reaching positive implications for practice, for the practitioner and patient relationship. There are many challenges to building relationships with people with learning disabilities but through mindfulness, presence and authenticity, the practitioner can meet these challenges with confidence. There are, however, additional qualities and skills in developing positive relationships with people with learning disabilities and these will be explored in the next section.

Scenario

Kate is a lady with learning disabilities and talks about building positive relationships.

Kate interviewed and employed Louisa as her Personal Assistant. Kate likes her PA because she likes her attitude towards her. It is supportive and Louisa expresses an interest in learning from Kate. They will go out for coffee and chat through Louisa's role. Louisa checks and asks Kate for feedback regularly about how she is doing and Kate likes this. It gives her a sense of control and that she is in charge. Kate would describe their relationship as relaxed and calm. Kate thinks that Louisa is sensitive to her needs, she smiles and is engaging. Occasionally she will hug her, hold hands or link arms. If people in Kate's environment are pleasant, polite and warm towards her, this will make Kate feel good and safe – she feels part of her community. One of the most important things for Kate is the need for people to really listen, spending time and talking things through with her. If people do not listen to Kate, she feels disempowered and becomes very uncomfortable. Kate said that trust is very important. Trust makes Kate feel in control, relaxed, she feels respected and like a person. Kate likes to be reassured. If Kate had to go into hospital this is the advice she would give:

- A visit prior to admission would be useful for Kate to plan ahead.
- Talk things through and especially explain procedures, explain what is likely to happen.

- Be friendly and approachable.
- Be patient and listen to what Kate has to say or be aware of how she feels.
- Promote comfort and be at ease, be comfortable around Kate.
- Help Kate overcome any fear or anxiety, ensure that she feels safe.
- Contact Kate's other PA and/or other people that know her.
- If possible, stay with Kate.
- Check with Kate if it is OK to share information about Kate's health needs with other people.
- Can you recognise any of Rogers' core conditions or Egan's 'micro-skills' in Kate's story? What are they?
- What skills is Louisa using in her relationship with Kate?
- Reflect on how you can promote Kate's advice when she is admitted into hospital.

SELF-AWARENESS, THERAPEUTIC USE OF SELF AND REFLECTIVE PRACTICE

There has been a steady interest in nursing literature about the concept of self-awareness and the role of the 'therapeutic use of self', its application to nursing and the impact on the nurse–client relationship (Cumbie, 2001; Freshwater, 2002; Stickley and Freshwater, 2002; Kwaitek et al., 2005; Jack and Smith, 2007; and Jack and Miller, 2008). What this body of literature suggests is that to be self-aware is an integral concept that defines nurses' therapeutic interactions with patients/clients, their families and members of the multi-disciplinary team. To be self-aware, learning more about ourselves, our attributions, values and attitudes, our strength and limitations, our thoughts, feelings and behaviours (Kwaitek et al., 2005) and how they impact on our relationships with clients is considered to be an essential ethical position to take. Humanistic and holistic nursing care hinges on the practitioner consciously knowing themselves, and to care for people requires a sophisticated degree of knowing who we are (Burnard, 1997). Our value base, attitudes and beliefs about people with learning disabilities will be reflected in how we communicate, interact and care for them. If we are aware of our personal attributes we are then in a stronger position to regard people with learning disabilities as people first, regardless of their behaviours, diagnoses or labels. This section will explore the concept of self-awareness and will discuss the Johari Window (Luft, 1969) and the importance of promoting an ethos of reflective practice as two frameworks to facilitate a better understanding of who we are.

Kwaitek et al. (2005) suggest that the 'therapeutic self' is a process of evaluating the consequences of our characteristics on others and the extent this brings about new learning and awareness. Rowe (1999) examined the components of the 'self' and articulated that a common theme among theorists of self-development is the idea of the public or open self which is seen by others and the private or closed self which is internal and not seen by others. This resonates with Luft's model of exploring aspects of the self (1969) and will be explored later. Cumbie (2001) recognises the importance of the therapeutic use of self and discusses this in the context of a philosophical perspective of the art of humanistic nursing. Immersing oneself completely into the phenomenology of caring, knowing one's subjective experiences and using the self as a resource in the professional relationship has the potential to rejuvenate the core principles of the therapeutic nature of nursing or, as Stickley and Freshwater (2002) state, stimulate a 're-enchantment' with them. A corollary of transpersonal care and by default self-awareness is that not only does the client benefit but the process is also therapeutic for the practitioner. The practitioner grows by being in touch with the self and the self within relationships.

In analysing self-awareness, there is an assumption that learning to use oneself therapeutically is relatively straightforward and that there are only positive outcomes for the client and the practitioner. Rowe (1999) warns that gaining more insight into ourselves can be painful and we may not like what we discover about ourselves. Kwaitek et al. (2005) highlight that working therapeutically can take its toll and can be demanding and challenging. Acting as if one is busy and not making time to engage with clients are natural defences against potential feelings of discomfort in the practitioner–patient relationship and dealing with feelings from clients can be difficult to manage (Jack and Smith, 2007). A further implication is that the art of nursing – that is the therapeutic, humanistic domain of caring – is being eroded where nursing functions in an increasingly bureaucratic, outcomes driven, fiscal savings and depersonalised service (Stickley and Freshwater, 2002). Being self-aware, empathic and authentic are often regarded as 'low visibility functions' (Brown and Fowler, cited in Jack and Miller, 2008) and consequently can be criticised because the practitioner is not detached, aloof or objective (Cumbie, 2001).

The Johari Window

The Johari Window (Figure 6.1) is a model for exploring and understanding self-awareness, personal development, interpersonal relationships, group dynamics and team development. It was first developed by Joseph Luft and Harry Ingham in the 1950s. It is also known as a feedback/disclosure model of self-awareness. The main principle is that the model explores the self – feelings, thoughts, motivation, attitudes, experience and skills – from four

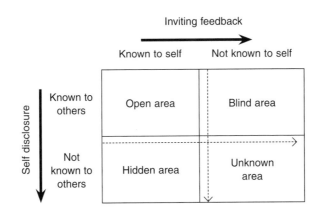

FIGURE 6.1   *The Johari Window (Luft, 1969)*

perspectives and is particularly relevant due to emphasis on and influence of behaviour, empathy, cooperation, interpersonal and inter-group development. Each perspective is known as a quadrant or area. Each area is examined in terms of whether thoughts and feelings are known or unknown to the person and known or unknown to others (within a team for example). Each area is known as *open* (known to self and known to others), *hidden* (known to self but not known to others) *blind* (not known to self but known to others) and *unknown* (not known to self and not known to others). When we learn more about ourselves through the processes of self-disclosure and inviting feedback the sizes of each area will change. For example, if I ask for and receive feedback about aspects of my behaviour or performance and if I reveal more of my hidden self to team members, then my open area will increase in size, my unknown area will shrink, and this will lead to a greater understanding of myself and others. There is an element of risk here because we have to trust others when listening to feedback and disclosing information about ourselves and what we hear may be painful (Jack and Smith, 2007). Giving feedback has to be honest, positive and affirming as the other person may not be aware of an aspect of their personality or behaviour and the impact it may have on clients and team members.

The ability to invite and receive feedback and to self-disclose and thus create opportunities to learn more about ourselves will depend on the interpersonal relationships of team members, and the overt culture of the working environment of the team. A team member is more likely to have a heightened sense of self-awareness if a team promotes a learning environment, encourages a sharing of different subjective points of view about nursing practice, and reflects on their individual and team performances. If the

Johari Window is embedded in a tradition of reflective practice then indi-viduals and teams are in a stronger position to learn more about themselves and each other. Self-awareness is a key factor of reflective practice (Horton-Deutsch and Sherwood, 2008) and a practitioner is more able to learn from experience if they have a structure to work to.

Reflection Point 17

Write notes about the learning philosophy of your team. Does it encourage the sharing of personal reflections?

Evaluate how easy or difficult it is for you and your team to receive and give feedback to colleagues. How could this be improved?

Evaluate how easy or difficult it is for you and your team to self-disclose. How could this be improved?

If you and your team provide care to a person with a learning disability, do you evaluate, record and learn from the care provided? How could this be improved?

Reflective Practice

There is not scope in this chapter to detail reflective practice (read Gibbs, 1988; Driscoll, 1994/2007; Johns, 1998; Burns and Bulman, 2000) other than to outline the relationship between reflective practice and self-awareness. A practitioner who is reflective is more likely to meet the needs of the client, more able to be genuine, empathic and warm and, therefore, more likely to apply Rogers' core conditions of the therapeutic relationship (Kwaitek et al., 2005). Reflection involves an exploration of one's feelings as well as the cognitive skills of describing, analysing, synthesising and evaluating experiences. An outcome of being a reflective practitioner is the increased ability to be competent in transpersonal caring and to manage one's emotions rather than be overtaken by them. When caring for a person with a learning disability, it is worth reflecting on how your values, attitudes and biases influence your approach and to reflect on your application of Rogers' (1957) three core conditions and Egan's (2007) micro-skills of attending and listening. Through reflective exploration you can promote partnerships that are based on sound ethical decision making, increase your involvement with clients and consider skilled and timely interventions. For example, knowing when to touch someone therapeutically (Gale and Hegarty, 2000), when and how to listen and give time (Gardner and Smyly, 1997), and when to communicate with and gather important information from significant carers so as to promote consistency of care between hospital and home (Gibbs et al., 2008).

PROMOTING SELF-ESTEEM IN PEOPLE WITH LEARNING DISABILITIES

From the ideas discussed in this chapter, it is assumed that becoming more self-aware, getting to know yourself better and learning to be reflective enables the practitioner to become more effective in the art of transpersonal care and that there are practical benefits to clients. It can also be assumed that building a positive, therapeutic relationship with a person with a learning disability raises their self-esteem, self-worth and confidence and helps them feel better about themselves. In essence, the attributes of the self-aware practitioner not only raise the health and well-being of the client but also enhance the health, well-being and self-esteem of the practitioner (Freshwater, 2002).

Self-esteem is often defined in terms of a personal evaluation of who we are as a person. Self-esteem tends to be regarded as an image of the self, how we feel about ourselves, our opinions and the value we place on ourselves as people (Fennell, 1999; Freshwater, 2002). This is consistent with Coopersmiths's reference to self-esteem where he asserts: 'self-esteem is a personal judgement of worthiness that is expressed in the attitudes the individual holds' (1967, cited in Burns, 1982: 6). This personal judgement of worthiness can be regarded as high or low. Having high self-esteem reflects a degree of self-confidence, self-worth and self-acceptance or self-regard. Low self-esteem can be perceived as a relentless and enduring poor and negative self-image. A person with low esteem will focus upon their weaknesses and differences rather than their strengths and abilities (Whelan et al., 2007). People with low self-esteem will feel inferior to others, will have many moments of self-doubt, be self-critical and think of themselves as unworthy and not entitled to positive experiences. These feelings of low self-worth tend to come from negative personal life experiences and from harmful messages they have received about the kind of person they are. In effect, negative self-beliefs are the keystone to low self-esteem (Fennell, 1999).

It has been suggested that people with learning disabilities have had poor life experiences, being subjected to marginalisation, prejudice and discrimination, abuse, lack of friendships, and having a constant sense of failure and incompetence (Caine and Hatton, 1998). They often perceive their own life events differently from their peers for example, progressing through their development milestones differently within the family, poor educational experiences, lack of opportunities for intimate relationships, and little chance of meaningful employment (Whelan et al., 2007). Additionally, many people seem to lack the social, interpersonal and coping skills necessary to deal with everyday life. It is not unusual for people with learning disabilities to be negatively labelled by society as a group who are less socially valued and, therefore, they are treated and related to differently, often negatively. People with learning disabilities then will generally have lower self-esteem compared to the general population (Thomson and McKenzie, 2005).

It would be reasonable to assume that one's relationship with society greatly influences a person's self-esteem. If a person with a learning disability is valued, recognised and shown positive regard then that person is more likely to consider themselves worthy and, accordingly, will begin to have a more positive sense of their own worth. It is important, therefore, for practitioners to think about how they can raise the self-esteem of people with learning disabilities so that they can begin to realise their own personal power. Equally, it is important that practitioners consider and look after their own esteem needs. Looking after oneself and meeting your own esteem needs in practice is important and protects against burnout. Failure to do so could result in practitioners raising their own self-esteem at the expense of the clients they are interacting with (Mosley, 1994).

Reflection Point 18

It has been argued that Person Centred Planning enables people with learning disabilities to make their own decisions and to have a clearer sense of direction in their lives. This in turn promotes the self-worth and esteem needs of people (Duffy and Smith, 2008). Person centred practice has the potential to empower people and enable them to have their human rights respected. It also facilitates and promotes independence, choice and inclusive practice (*Valuing People*, DH, 2001).

Reflect on your's and your team's attitudes towards people with learning disabilities. Do you promote their rights, independence and choices? What influence do you have in these areas of their lives? How could these areas be improved when accessing health or social care environments?

Do you encourage and promote inclusive practice? How could this be improved?

How do you know if a person with a learning disability has high or low self-esteem?

What could you and your team do to improve their self-esteem?

CONCLUSION

This chapter has explored Rogers' core conditions of congruence, unconditional positive regard and empathy (1957) and considered their application
to people with learning disabilities through the practitioners' verbal, non-
verbal and para-verbal behaviour. Egan (2007) advocated breaking interpersonal
skills down into individual 'micro-skills' as a framework to learning the key
skills of attending and listening. It has been emphasised that active listening
is vital to developing trust and rapport with clients which, in turn, promotes
a mutually respected relationship where the client functions in a climate of
self-worth and self-determination. Competent and skilled listening also
demonstrates that the practitioner wishes to encourage the client to express
themselves, to express their rights and choices and, wherever possible,
acknowledging and endorsing inclusive practice. This chapter has also
emphasised the necessity of developing self-awareness, how to use oneself
in the therapeutic relationship and the value of reflective practice.
Combining and practicing all of these skills, values and approaches has the
potential to promote self-esteem in people with learning disabilities. Feeling
good about yourself contributes to the healing process and creates a mutually conducive working environment whereby people can have positive
experiences when they go into hospital or need to access other primary
care workers.

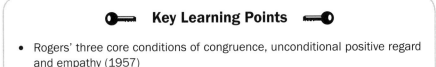

Key Learning Points

- Rogers' three core conditions of congruence, unconditional positive regard
  and empathy (1957)
- Egan's SOLER framework for learning the micro-skills of attending and lis-
  tening (2007)
- The value of self-awareness and the therapeutic use of self
- The Johari Window (Luft, 1969). A model of developing self-awareness
- Enhancing reflective practice when building positive relationships with
  people with learning disabilities
- Promoting self-esteem.

REFERENCES

Boudreau, J.D., Cassell, E. and Fuks, A. (2009) 'Preparing medical students to become
    attentive listeners', *Medical Teacher,* 31 (1): 22–9.
Bryant, L. (2009) 'The art of active listening', *Practice Nurse,* 37 (6): 49–52.
Burnard, P. (1997) *Know Yourself: Self Awareness Activities for Nurses and Other Health
    Professionals.* London: Whurr Publishers.

Burns, R.B. (1982) *Self Concept Development and Education*. London: Holt, Rinehart and Winston.

Burns, S. and Bulman, C. (2000) *Reflective Practice in Nursing: The Growth of the Professional Practitioner*, Oxford: Blackwell Science.

Caine, A. and Hatton, C. (1998) 'Working with people with mental health problems', in E. Emerson, C. Hatton, J. Bromley and A. Caine (eds), *Clinical Psychology and People with Intellectual Disabilities*. Chichester: John Wiley and Sons Ltd.

Chambers, S. (2003) 'Use of non-verbal communication skills to improve nursing care', *British Journal of Nursing*, 12 (14): 874–8.

Cumbie, S.A. (2001) 'The integration of mind–body–soul and the practice of humanistic nursing', *Holistic Nursing Practice*, 15 (3): 56–62.

Department of Health (2001) *Valuing People: A Strategy for People with Learning Disabilities in the 21st Century*. London: Department of Health.

Driscoll, J. (1994) 'Reflective practice for practice', *Senior Nurse*, 13 (7): 47–50.

Driscoll, J. (2007) *Practicing Clinical Supervision: A Reflective Approach for Healthcare Professionals*. Edinburgh: Bailliere Tindall.

Duffy, S. and Smith, S. (2008) 'Person centred partnerships', in J. Thompson, J. Kilbane and H. Sanderson (eds), *Person Centred Practice for Professionals*. Maidenhead: Open University Press.

Egan, G. (2007) *The Skilled Helper: A Problem-management and Opportunity-development Approach to Helping* (8th edn). Belmont, CA: Thomson Brooks/Cole.

Fennell, M. (1999) *Overcoming Low Self Esteem. A Self-help Guide using Cognitive Behavioural Techniques*. London: Constable and Robinson Ltd.

Fitzsimmons, J. and Barr, O. (1997) 'A review of the reported attitudes of health and social care professionals towards people with learning disabilities', *Journal of Intellectual Disabilities*, 1 (2): 57–64.

Freshwater, D. (2002) 'The therapeutic use of the nursing self', in D. Freshwater (ed.), *Therapeutic Nursing*. London: Sage.

Gale, E. and Hegarty, J.R. (2000) 'The use of touch in caring for people with learning disabilities', *British Journal of Developmental Disabilities*, 46 (2): 97–108.

Gardner, A. and Smyly, S.R. (1997) 'How do we stop "doing" and start listening: responding to the emotional needs of people with learning disabilities', *British Journal of Learning Disabilities*, 25: 26–9.

Gibbs, G. (1988) *Learning by Doing: A Guide to Teaching and Learning Methods*. Oxford: Oxford Brookes University.

Gibbs, S., Brown, M.J. and Muir, W.J. (2008) 'The experience of adults with intellectual disabilities and their carers in general hospitals: a focus group study', *Journal of Intellectual Disability Research*, 52 (12): 1061–77.

Horton-Deutsch, S. and Sherwood, G. (2008) 'Reflection: an educational strategy to develop emotionally-competent nurse leaders', *Journal of Nursing Management*. 16: 946–54.

Jack, K. and Miller, E. (2008) 'Exploring self-awareness in mental health practice', *Mental Health Practice*, 12 (3): 31–5.

Jack, K. and Smith, A. (2007) 'Promoting self awareness in nurses to improve nursing practice', *Nursing Standard*, 21 (32): 47–52.

Johns, C. (1998) 'Opening the doors of perception', in C. Johns and D. Freshwater (eds), *Transforming Nursing Through Reflective Practice*. Oxford: Blackwell Science.

Kwaitek, E., McKenzie, K. and Loads, D. (2005) 'Self-awareness and reflection: exploring the "therapeutic use of self"', *Learning Disability Practice*, 8 (3): 27–31.

Luft, J. (1969) *On Human Interaction*. Palo Alto, CA: National Press.

McNaughton, D., Hamlin, D., McCarthy, J., Head-Reeves, D. and Schreiner, M. (2008) 'Learning to listen. Teaching an active listening strategy to preservice education professionals', *Topics in Early Childhood Special Education*, 27 (4): 223–31.

Mosley J. (1994) *You Choose*. London: LDA.

Rogers, C.R. (1957) 'The necessary and sufficient conditions of therapeutic personality change', *Journal of Consulting Psychology*, 21: 95–103.

Rowe, J. (1999) 'Self awareness: improving nurse-client interactions', *Nursing Standard*, 14 (8): 37–40.

Stickley, T. and Freshwater, D. (2002) 'The art of loving and the therapeutic relationship', *Nursing Inquiry*, 9 (4): 250–6.

Thomas, D. and Woods, H. (2003) *Working with People with Learning Disabilities – Theory and Practice*. London: Jessica Kingsley Publishers.

Thomson, R. and McKenzie, K. (2005) 'What people with a learning disability understand and feel about having a learning disability', *Learning Disability Practice*, 8 (6): 28–32.

Whelan, A., Haywood, P. and Galloway, S. (2007) 'Low self esteem: cognitive behaviour therapy', *British Journal of Learning Disabilities*, 35: 125–30.

7 PROMOTING EFFECTIVE COMMUNICATION

Robert Pardoe

INTRODUCTION

> No one would talk much in society, if he knew how often he misunderstood others. (JW van Goethe. 1749–1832)

Goethe here is relating verbal communication – 'talk' – to the world in general (in Goethe's time 'he' referred to both men and women). The opportunity for misunderstanding the spoken word is significantly enhanced when the communication needs of people with learning disabilities are taken into account. This chapter intends to enhance the reader's understanding of how people with a range of learning disabilities experience and perceive communication. First, the importance of communication in terms of the place it plays in the lives of all of us will be identified and, in so doing, the possible consequences of not being able to engage in mainstream communication will be exposed. Second, the intention is to highlight the philosophy of 'Total Communication' as a starting point for working with people with learning disabilities. Third, there will be an examination of the sort of communication difficulties that are commonly experienced by people with learning disabilities and the strategies that might be employed to help overcome those difficulties. Finally, the use of Alternative and Augmentative communication will be explored in order to identify a range of tools and techniques which are available (both low and high tech) to promote opportunities that can be afforded to people with learning disabilities to enhance and extend their communication abilities.

WHAT IS COMMUNICATION?

According to Bunning, 'Communication is the conduit between the individual and the world. It is the very cornerstone of identity formation, social engagement and human relationships' (2009: 46). Bunning (2009) ascribes highly significant value to communication here. Its role in forming identity and in being the cornerstone of human relationships suggests that, if someone's ability to communicate in a similar way to which the world generally communicates is either significantly limited or absent, then their whole self-identity is put at risk. Communication is the door through which access to self-knowledge, self-worth and self-esteem is made available. People for whom communication is a challenge are therefore potentially deprived of these 'cornerstone' developmental opportunities, alongside a whole lot of other privations which will become apparent. The importance, therefore, of creating opportunities for people to discover ways in which they can both express and receive communication cannot be overstated. If Bunning is right in her contention then it is paramount that carers, families and others who seek to build relationships with people with learning disabilities are able to draw on a range of strategies and techniques that may enable, among other things, important choices to be made by the person, value and respect to be given to the person, and control and power to be shared with the person. *Valuing People* (DH, 2001) and the follow up White Paper *Valuing People Now* (DH, 2009) both identify four key principles that should be at the heart of all services for people with learning disabilities. These are facilitating choice, independence, social inclusion and civil rights. The Equalities Act (2010) is clear in its identification of the need for reasonable adjustments to be made in all areas of employment, buying and renting land, and using services and amenities so that people with a disability are not discriminated against. The way this has been interpreted has obviously emphasised physical access, but it also relates very clearly to the need for accessible communication also to be considered. The Human Rights Act (1998), Article 10: Freedom of Expression has additional guidance attached to it (Department of Constitutional Affairs, 2006) which supports the use of communication methods that are most natural and apposite for individuals in order for communication to be achieved. All these government drivers and policy directives clearly confirm the part that effective communication can play in dramatically enhancing the lives and experiences of people with learning disabilities.

It is important to remember that, because the descriptor of learning disabilities covers a wide range of people, then the nature and range of communication difficulties will be similarly wide. As a result, this brief exploration offers some general principles to be followed, and does not provide a blueprint for meeting the individual communication needs of all those people who are identified under the umbrella of learning disabilities.

TOTAL COMMUNICATION

The concept of 'total communication' was originally conceived as a communication approach in relation to the deaf community by David Denton and then further developed by Roy Holcomb at the Maryland School for the Deaf (Schlesinger, 1986).

> A communication philosophy – not a communication method and not at all a teaching method ... Total Communication is an approach to create a successful and equal communication between human beings with different language perception and/or production. To use Total Communication amounts to a willingness to use all available means in order to understand and be understood. (Hansen, 1980: 22)

While there is no evidence to support such a stance, it would be easy to rank different communication methods in a sort of hierarchy in which spoken and written language is seen as more significant and important than, say, signs or symbols. Clearly, most of us are familiar with and use the spoken word in our everyday lives with no pause for thought at all. Total Communication asks us to do exactly that: *to pause for thought* before we assume that our preferred method of communication is also shared by the person we are in communication with. There is no hierarchy within this philosophy. All forms of communication have value and each might be appropriate in particular circumstances and for particular individuals. Indeed, the communication needs of some people with learning disabilities might be such that the use of pre-verbal/pre-intentional communication or early gestures – such as touch, eye-contact, smiles and other significant facial gestures, pointing or indicating – might be the most appropriate form of contact and communication (Saltford SaLT Department, 2001). This might sound like 'baby talk' and, indeed the very nature of it is taken from the way babies and young children are introduced to the world of talk and language, but it is attempting to acknowledge where the person is with their language development and the need for these stages of communication to be worked through in order to develop the communicative abilities of the person. There are ways of providing the same pre-verbal/pre-intentional experiences without the accompanying 'coochy-coos'.

Total Communication is thus concerned with exploring all aspects of communication to discover what best works for a person. Rather than imposing one's own preferred technique and maintaining that technique despite its inadequacies, Total Communication asks us to be innovative and creative, and to look at all the alternative ways in which messages can be sent and received and employ the most effective approach for the person we are working with. This is an empathic and valuing intervention rather than one which is controlling and overpowering.

A BASIC MODEL OF COMMUNICATION

The basic components of communication can be summed up for our purposes in a simple model which identifies two components: expression and understanding. Expression refers to a person's ability to make themselves understood: to communicate needs and desires, to share feelings and emotions, to initiate and terminate engagements/encounters. Understanding refers to a person's ability to receive those same expressed messages from the other person. People with learning disabilities can and often do encounter problems and challenges with both these components. First of all the problems and challenges of understanding will be explored.

Barriers to Understanding

Clearly, as already alluded to, some people with learning disabilities will have such extreme communication needs that understanding any spoken word is difficult because they haven't yet begun (or had the opportunities) to develop the foundation skills of communication. Attempting to gain their understanding through the spoken word is likely to be fruitless and alternative approaches to enabling them to engage with what is happening to them will need to be found. The use of Alternative and Augmentative Communication strategies is likely to be important here and these strategies are explored later on in this chapter. Other people with learning disabilities might be able to receive some fairly complex ideas through the spoken word but will not necessarily be able to decode some of the additional components that accompany such conversations, such as sarcasm or the use of metaphor. In addition, it is sometimes easy to overestimate a person's understanding or receptive language skills because they are able to disguise their limitations in a variety of ways. For instance, people will use non-verbal cues and familiarity with routine (and the behaviours that accompany them) to make sense of events without necessarily understanding the words that are spoken at the time.

Scenario

Imagine a residential setting and lunch is just about to be served. A member of staff enters the lounge and announces that lunch is about to be dished up. It might only require one person (indeed it might even be a member of staff who has been sitting down) to get up immediately and walk towards the dining room for everyone present to 'pick up the message' and do likewise. It would be inappropriate to ascribe understanding of the phrase 'lunch is about to be dished up' to all those that picked up the message through other means (e.g. the fact that they were hungry, the fact that this happens about this time every day, the fact that everyone else was getting up, so something must be happening). It is important not to assume understanding simply on that sort of evidence.

This is a very simple example, but there are lots of occasions in which it is possible for a person with a learning disability to respond to a verbal request or suggestion appropriately because they have understood it through cues other than verbal ones. Therefore, if we want to enhance our abilities to make ourselves understood more effectively by the people we support, we need to use strategies alongside verbal means to strengthen the messages that we want to communicate. Total Communication would suggest looking at the following areas for consideration:

Use short straightforward sentences. For example, it is easy to construct a fairly long, rambling sentence with a number of different clauses in it when we try to communicate verbally: 'I am not here tomorrow because I am going on holiday next weekend and I need to book my train journey because otherwise I won't get the cheapest deal on the tickets.' It is likely to be difficult to hold onto all the ideas held in this sentence. It might be better delivered in four shorter sentences with the most important message delivered last: 'I am going on holiday next week. I need to book my train journey. The tickets are cheaper if I get them soon. So I am not here tomorrow'.

Maintain consistent use of vocabulary. For example, Granny, Gran, Nanny, Nan, Grandma, Grandmother, Grandparent (or any number of special family diminutives) are all ways of describing the mother of one's father or mother. Only one of them is likely to be right for any of us. While most of us can appreciate the rich diversity of vocabulary that characterises the English language, employing such diversity is unlikely to aid understanding for someone whose receptive understanding is limited. In addition to this, cultural diversity adds another dimension to the use of vocabulary and needs careful consideration when trying to support people with learning disabilities to engage with their worlds.

Emphasise important words. This could be done by indicating the object or direction, by using pictures or photographs, actually handling the object being referred to, or by using signs and symbols. This will be explored in more detail when Alternative and Augmentative methods of communication are explored.

Slow your speech (but don't lose the rhythm). Try to keep the natural rhythm and tone of your voice, but just allow more time for the information to be processed between sentences. If it is too unnaturally slow then the other non-verbal cues that accompany speech will be corrupted and these cues are just as important, if not more so, for a clear understanding of the message to be received.

Avoid abstract concepts and ideas. Concepts of time are often difficult to convey. Diaries or daily logs can assist here. Metaphors are sometimes very difficult for someone who takes a literal view of the spoken word (for example someone on the autistic spectrum). Phrases like, 'Hop in and I'll drop you off at the end of the road', or 'You mustn't run before you can walk' will not necessarily communicate the message in the way wanted.

After that brief examination of some of the challenges people face with regard to understanding communication, the difficulties faced with regard to expression will now be explored.

BARRIERS TO EXPRESSION

First, any difficulty a person has with understanding communication is quite possibly going to lead to problems with expression (Skelhorn and Williams, 2008). These difficulties might manifest themselves in a variety of ways. A person might have developed a range of 'stock' phrases, for example: 'Good morning …what a lovely day it is'; 'I am going on holiday, I am'. These are expressed perfectly clearly and articulately but they are used in a large variety of situations, many of which are not entirely appropriate for their use. In other words, they are being used for a different purpose than the actual content of the message might be considered to convey. It could be to deal with anxiety, as a means of engaging in social contact, or to meet any number of other idiosyncratic needs which cannot be met otherwise. Therefore, as with some of the difficulties with understanding it is important not to misinterpret or overestimate someone's expressive ability simply on the basis of the language they choose to use. The involvement of a speech and language therapist (with learning disabilities expertise) here might enable a much more detailed and thorough assessment of the abilities a person has with regard to communication.

Furthermore, some people for whom the spoken word is not their chosen form of communication might indulge in a rich range of alternative behaviours to express their needs and to maintain some control over what happens to them. Osgood (2004) uses the phrase 'exotic' communication to describe this particular means of expression: others might describe the behaviours as challenging. Certainly, one very legitimate way of explaining such events is supplied by Osgood:

> Problem behaviour/challenging behaviour/exotic communication/whatever we call the phenomena … these events are simply adaptive behaviours given the limitations of the environment, the unusual learning history and the skills of the person … They're telling us somehow we're not meeting the person's needs. (2004: 2)

Such forms of expression clearly have a part to play in enabling some people to gain some control of their lives and to enable them to make their needs met. Therefore, it seems appropriate to include this explanation for some challenging behaviours in a section which is concerned with expressive communication.

Scenario

Imagine a hospital setting. A member of staff walks into the room eating a sandwich. There is a patient with learning disabilities sitting down who is feeling hungry but does not have the communication skills to request a sandwich for himself, nor the opportunity or skills to make it himself. Seeing the sandwich gives him the idea that there is the possibility of food being immediately available. He starts to bang his hand on the arm of his wheelchair and to rock his head back and forth, hitting his head on the side of the chair. The member of staff interprets the behaviour as a request for something to eat and reassures the person that this will be done. As a result of the reassurance and the soon-to-be-made sandwich, the service user stops the behaviour.

This is a classic behavioural transaction. It is not saying that this is the right intervention. Unpacking all the theories of learning and ideas related to how challenging behaviours (or exotic communication) are developed and maintained is not for this text (see Emerson, 2003, for a much more detailed examination of these ideas). This is simply to illustrate the fact that some people use a range of complex behaviours as a means of expression to get their needs met much more effectively sometimes than would be the case otherwise.

In addition to this there might be other difficulties with expression to do with articulation and fluency. A learning disability might be accompanied by a difficulty in the physical manipulation of the mouth and jaw which renders the spoken word difficult to formulate in a way which is accessible to a new listener. Some forms of Cerebral Palsy, for instance, can result in such difficulties. Stammering and other difficulties with fluency can also manifest themselves in some people with learning disabilities and make expressive language much more complicated both to deliver and to receive.

In order to enhance the communicative abilities of people with learning disabilities there are a number of strategies, again drawn from the philosophy of Total Communication, which could be employed:

Encourage people to use the form of communication that best works for them. Don't impose a preferred form of communication but be prepared to work with and enable a person to use the technique with which they are most comfortable. This does not mean that you should not try, at other times, to extend their range of communication abilities. After all, the more skills one has, the more opportunity one will have to integrate and engage with a wider group of people.

Always be prepared to give time to the speaker. The more time you have to enable a person to find their own way to express needs and wishes, the more likely you are to get their story, and not your own or someone else's interpretation of 'their story'. Also, giving time will enable someone with a stutter or a stammer to complete their account without feeling under pressure (which generally exacerbates the stammer or stutter). It is among the most generous acts to allow people space to tell their stories, but it can also be a highly rewarding experience too. It is a great way to communicate value to someone, to let them know that you are really listening to them by giving them time to complete their conversations and resisting the temptation to edit or reinterpret their words in order to save you time. This is an important matter to consider before you embark on any meaningful conversation with someone in this situation.

Accept the communication without judgement. It would be very easy to seek to correct an inarticulate or poorly constructed piece of communication. However, if the message was understood then this would be time not well spent. Just accept it in the way it was delivered and move on.

Make judicious use of questioning. Open questions rather than closed questions are likely to be more effective in supporting someone to express themselves. For instance, if a person is unable to think of the right word for an object, then asking questions which narrow down the range of areas in which the object might be used is likely to be more helpful in identifying it, than simply attempting to guess. In addition, when trying to enable a person to tell their story, asking questions which allow for choice and diversity in response are more helpful – and indeed more likely to illicit more truthful accounts – than closed or leading questions which demand a single word reply or a particular response.

Using visual aids. There are a number of commercial strategies and approaches to this that will be referred to in a little more detail later on, but the simple use of pictures or objects of reference (Ockelford, 2002) can really enhance and enrich the communicative abilities of a person with a learning disability, particularly if the pictures are photographs taken of real objects and places in the person's life (the local pub, the local post office, their own mug, bedroom, etc.).

Reflection Point 19

Think of a situation in which you are working with a patient or service user with a learning disability.

What challenges have you experienced in terms of being able to make yourself understood and what ideas might you now use to make yourself more easily understood?

What challenges have they experienced in terms of being able to make themselves understood to you and what ideas might you now use to enable them to make themselves more easily understood?

This completes the second section of this chapter in which a very simple model of communication has been identified and then some of the barriers to understanding and expressing communications and some strategies for overcoming those barriers have been explored. Alternative and Augmentative Communication strategies will now be examined in a little more detail and resources related to them will be highlighted.

ALTERNATIVE AND AUGMENTATIVE COMMUNICATION STRATEGIES

People for whom verbal communication is not their preferred mode of interaction or for whom verbal communication is difficult to understand, can sometimes be offered either an alternative communications strategy or a strategy which augments their sometimes limited verbal skills. These come in a range of guises, some with considerable commercial energy attached to them. They all offer techniques and ideas for enhancing the communicative ability of the person and/or enhancing the ability of others to communicate with the person. In this section, a number of these ideas will be identified and described, alongside details of how to contact the commercial organisations who are responsible for them. There are no particular recommendations being given here, nor any hierarchy of preference in the way they are being presented. All these strategies have made a contribution to enriching the communicative abilities of people with learning disabilities and therefore might be useful to employ in any of the situations in which the reader might find themselves.

Intensive Interaction

This particular communication strategy was developed by a group of staff working in a long-stay hospital who were caring for a group of children with severe learning disabilities (Nind and Hewitt, 1994, 2001). They were struggling to engage with and get to know them and wanted an approach that would allow the service user and the staff member (known under the strategy as the communication partner) to enjoy being in each other's company. It is based on a model of caregiver–infant interaction, and works by focussing on the quality of everyday interactions. It is a method of engagement which tries to respond to what the person with learning disabilities brings to an interaction, allowing them to take the lead and share fully in the give and take that characterises most episodes of effective communication. Giving space for the person to take control of the interaction is both empowering and valuing. While Intensive Interaction can be part of a fairly formal therapeutic intervention strategy, the principles of following the communicative lead of the person and encouraging the sharing of the communicative space with the person with learning disabilities can be explored and practised in any setting. It is a really helpful way for putting the person at the centre of any interaction and a way of letting them know that they are important and that they matter in whatever situation they are in. For further information visit http://www.intensiveinteraction.co.uk/ and http://www.phoebecaldwell.co.uk/.

Signing Systems

There are a number of signing systems that have been used to assist people with learning disabilities to both express and receive communication. Most can be used in addition to the spoken word so that they support attempts to articulate even if it is indistinct. Three are identified here which have been used most regularly in the field of people with learning disabilities

The Makaton Vocabulary System

This is a very widely used approach which involves the use of signs, symbols and speech. The signs and symbols are derived from British Sign Language for deaf people and, in its first guise (early 1970s), it was intended to meet the needs of people with learning disabilities who were living in hospital and had an additional hearing loss. In its latest revision (1996) it has been updated to reflect both changes in the way services are provided for people with learning disabilities and the more multiculturally diverse and technologically advanced society that Britain has become. It has also been adapted for use in over forty different countries across the globe. It involves a core vocabulary of about 450 words, with an additional 7,000 words in the resource vocabulary. The intention is that carers or families should tailor the selection and use of vocabulary to the individual needs of the person so that it reflects their interests, daily activities and their environment. The individualised nature of this selection is one of the important features of this system. Clearly the fact that this is both a nationally and internationally recognised system makes it particularly appealing since service users who move about between services can expect that staff will be familiar with the system wherever the person finds themselves. The Makaton Organisation offers a full range of commercial resources to support the system as well as comprehensive training and updating for staff in its use.

Further information and advice can be obtained from the main Makaton website at http://www.makaton.org.

Paget Gorman Signing System

The Paget Gorman signing system was originated by Sir Richard Paget in the 1930s and then further developed by his wife (Lady Grace Paget) in collaboration with Dr Pierre Gorman. It is based on the idea that sign language is the original form of all speech and after many years of development and elaboration it now offers 'a grammatical sign system which reflects normal patterns of English and is used by many speech and language-impaired children, their parents, teachers, speech therapists and care staff' (Paget Gorman Sign System [PGSS], 2008). It provides a manual of 4,000 signs which, with additional affixes, gives signs to access the meaning of over 56,000 different words. The importance of accurate signing is emphasised (indeed it is equated with accurate pronunciation) and much focus is placed on the way one's hands and fingers are held and placed during signing. Fine motor coordination is a significant component of the system.

Further information and advice can be obtained from the main Paget Gorman Signing System website at http://www.pgss.org/.

SignAlong

SignAlong is a sign-supporting system based on British Sign Language designed to help children and adults with communication difficulties, mostly associated with learning disabilities, which is user-friendly for easy access. SignAlong empowers children and adults with impaired communication to understand and express their needs, choices and desires by providing vocabulary for life and learning. The SignAlong Group has researched and published the widest range of signs in Britain. These are drawn and described following a consistent method that enables users to access vocabulary according to need.

Further information and advice can be obtained from the main SignAlong website at http://www.signalong.org.uk/index.htm.

Strategies for Supporting and Augmenting Communication

In addition to formal signing systems, MacDonald (1998) identified a hierarchy of strategies for supporting and augmenting communication for people with learning disabilities. This suggests that the nearer the representation could be to reality the more effective the communicative quality of that representation. The hierarchy is represented in Table 7.1, with some examples of commercially available systems which reflect the levels in that hierarchy.

Reflection Point 20

Many accessible health information resources use photographs, pictures, line drawings, and easy words to support people with learning disabilities and improve their understanding of health and health interventions.

Spend some time reviewing the information leaflets that are used in your area of practice.

How effective are they for communicating with people for whom the written word is not their preferred method of communication?

Take at least one of them and think through how to make the information more accessible and more meaningful. Refer to some of the tools and techniques that were outlined in the final section of this chapter.

TABLE 7.1   *Hierarchies for Supporting Augmentative Communication*

---

1. Real Objects (clearly representational)

Using real objects such as a person giving you a real cup to get a drink. Real objects provide good communication reference for offering choices.
Tangible Symbols and Objects of Reference: further information and advice can be obtained from:
http://www.projectsalute.net/Learned/Learnedhtml/TangibleSymbols.html
http://www.ace-centre.org.uk/index.cfm?pageid=3CDC028A-3048-7290-FE7DEA7A0060EF46

2. Tactile Symbols

Tactile items can be used to offer choices, for example a piece of towelling to indicate having a bath.
Tangible Symbols and Objects of Reference: further information and advice can be obtained from:
http://www.projectsalute.net/Learned/Learnedhtml/TangibleSymbols.html
http://www.ace-centre.org.uk/index.cfm?pageid=3CDC028A-3048-7290-FE7DEA7A0060EF46

3. Photographs

Photographs of real items and people. Real photographs are often used in communication passports.
Picture Exchange Communication System (PECS): further information and advice can be obtained from the main PECS site at http://www.pecs.org.uk/general/what.htm
Communication Passports http://www.communicationpassports.org.uk/Home/

4. Miniatures of Real Objects

3D objects but much smaller. This means the person can have more of them to use and they are more transportable. But people need to learn to use them.
Tangible Symbols and Objects of Reference: further information and advice can be obtained from the following two sites:
http://www.totalcommunication.org.uk/objects-of-reference.html
http://www.ace-centre.org.uk/index.cfm?pageid=3CDC028A-3048-7290-FE7DEA7A0060EF46

5. Coloured Pictures

These may be photographs but could be very realistic drawings.
Picture Exchange Communication System (PECS): further information and advice can be obtained from the main PECS site at http://www.pecs.org.uk/general/what.htm

6. Line Drawings – Realistic

These have lost lots of the detail of the real thing but are still recognisable.
Scope have lots of examples of using different types of drawings to help improve communication.
http://www.scopevic.org.au/index.php/site/resources/communicationaids#ElectronicCommunicationDevices
There are a lot of strategies for this approach to enhancing communication: for further information about using symbols go to www.easyinfo.org.uk http://www.easyhealth.org.uk/

7. Line Drawings – Stylised

Stylised drawings are often abstract and have lost most if not all of their representational value.
For examples visit:
Widgit literacy symbols (formally Rebus): further information and advice can be obtained from the main Widgit site at http://www.widgit.com/symbols
Blissymbols: further information and advice can be obtained from the main Blissymbolics website at http://www.blissymbolics.us/

8. Written Words (abstract representation)

Clearly this relates to ordinary forms of the written word. To ensure the communication partner fully understands what an object or symbol means to an individual it is good practice to have the written word on or under the object or symbol to minimise confusion.

Based on MacDonald (1998)

CONCLUSION

In this chapter the profound significance of communication has been explored and the role it plays in giving value to a person with learning disabilities, developing self-esteem, empowerment and choice making. A very simple model for understanding communication has been put forward and the barriers both to expression and to understanding that might be faced by people with learning disabilities have been uncovered. Some techniques that should be used to enable people to overcome some of those barriers have also been highlighted. Finally, a number of alternative and augmentative communication strategies have also been described and details for obtaining further information have been identified. Building, maintaining and developing relationships (whether for a short-lived intervention or on the basis of a longer period of engagement) requires a real understanding of the specific individual communication needs of the person concerned. This chapter makes a sincere attempt to explore some general principles that can be applied to that task.

Reflection Point 21

Think about your own communication skills and identify a personal goal to achieve to improve how you communicate with people who have communication difficulties. Make this a SMART goal (see the Introduction chapter to review what a SMART goal is).

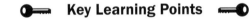 **Key Learning Points**

- Understanding the barriers to effective communication
- That everybody, regardless of disability, has communication strategies: practitioners need to learn these
- Effective communication needs to be person centred
- Accessible information is essential to support people's understanding of their health
- To enable effective communication practitioners have a responsibility for their own communication development.

REFERENCES

Bunning, K. (2009) 'Making sense of communication', in J. Pawlyn and S. Carnaby (eds), *Profound Intellectual and Multiple Disabilities: Nursing Complex Needs.* Chichester: Wiley Blackwell.

Department of Constitutional Affairs (2006) *A Guide to the Human Rights Act 1998* (3rd edn). London: Department of Constitutional Affairs.

Department of Health (2001) *Valuing People: A New Strategy for Learning Disability for the 21st Century*. London: Department of Health.

Department of Health (2009) *Valuing People Now – A New Three Year Strategy for People with Learning Disabilities*. London: Department of Health.

Emerson, E. (2003) *Challenging Behaviour: Analysis and Intervention in People with Severe Intellectual Disabilities* (2nd edn). Cambridge: Cambridge University Press.

Equalities Act (2010) London: HMSO.

Hansen, B. (1980) *Aspects of Deafness and Total Communication in Denmark*. Copenhagen: The Centre for Total Communication.

Human Rights Act (1998) London: HMSO.

MacDonald, A. (1998) 'Symbol Systems', in *Augmentative Communication In Practice: An Introduction*. Edinburgh: CALL Centre and Scottish Executive Education Department.

Nind, M. and Hewett, D. (1994) *Access to Communication: Developing the Basics of Communication with People with Severe Learning Difficulties through Intensive Interaction*. London: David Fulton.

Nind, M. and Hewett, D. (2001) *A Practical Guide to Intensive Interaction*. Kidderminster: British Institute of Learning Disabilities.

Ockelford, A. (2002) *Objects of Reference*. London: RNIB.

Osgood, T. (2004) *'Suits you Sir?': Challenging Behaviour in Learning Disability Services*. [online] Available from http://www.paradigm-uk.org/articles/Suits_you__challenging_behaviour_in_learning_disability_services/199/31.aspx, accessed 17.03.2011.

Paget Gorman Sign System (PGSS) (2008) *The Paget-Gorman Society*. [online] Available from http://www.pgss.org/manual/IntroPaget.html, Accessed on 04.06.10.

Saltford Speech and Language Therapy Department (SaLT) (2001) 'Communication model', in L. Skelhorn and K. Williams (2008), 'Communciation', cited in J. Thompson, J. Kilbane and H. Sanderson (eds), *Person Centred Practice for Professionals*. Maidenhead: Open University Press.

Schlesinger, H. (1986) 'Total communication in perspective' in D. Luterman (ed.), *Deafness in Perspective*. San Diego, CA: College-Hill Press.

Skelhorn, L. and Williams, K. (2008) 'Communciation', in J. Thompson, J. Kilbane and H. Sanderson (eds), *Person Centred Practice for Professionals*. Maidenhead: Open University Press.

8 HEALTH AND WELL-BEING

Matthew Godsell

INTRODUCTION

Over the last sixty years many people with learning disabilities have been resettled in the community from long-stay hospitals. They have joined a larger group of people with learning disabilities in the community that includes people living independently and people living with their families or other informal carers. Responsibility for their healthcare has been divided between two groups of practitioners. One group includes practitioners with specialised knowledge and the experience that they have gained from working with people with learning disabilities on a regular basis; the other group includes mainstream providers in primary and secondary care that may have limited or infrequent contact with people with learning disabilities. *Valuing People* established the principle that people with learning disabilities 'have the same right of access to mainstream services as the rest of the population' (DH, 2001: 6) and *Healthcare For All* (Michael Report, 2008) put a strong emphasis on the legislative framework that compelled the providers of services to make reasonable adjustments to support the delivery of equal treatment.

Providing more accessible services has been problematic. Nurses working in mainstream health services have reported that they lack confidence and do not have the background knowledge that they need to work with patients with learning disabilities (Backer et al., 2009). To overcome some of the problems that have impeded access, policy and best practice have provided the impetus for new partnerships and collaborative arrangements. Partnerships include the emergence of a new role for liaison nurses who work in hospitals to ensure the safety and well-being of people with learning disabilities by working with ward staff. Collaboration and a more consistent approach to the delivery of care have been promoted through the introduction of patient passports which convey vital information about an individual with learning disabilities to all of the practitioners that he or she might come into contact with.

Alongside these advances there have also been more pervasive changes in health and social care which have focussed on the use of evidence to support best practice. Developing an awareness of the range of evidence that supports innovation or an intervention requires more rigour than an approach that is reliant on tradition, intuition, or trial and error. Some professions insist that the decisions practitioners are compelled to take and the care that they deliver must incorporate reference to an appropriate and up-to-date evidence base. The *Standards of conduct, performance and ethics for nurses and midwives* produced by the Nursing and Midwifery Council (NMC) (2008) states that nurses and midwives must deliver care that is based on the 'best available evidence or practice' and that nurses and midwives need to ensure that any advice they give relating to healthcare products or services is evidence based.

This chapter will examine a range of ideas and developments that aim to improve the health of people with learning disabilities. The first section will examine a person's immediate needs when they enter a healthcare setting. The next section will begin to address some of the evidence for health inequalities and people with learning disabilities. The third section is called Evidence Based Practice. The material in this section will examine models that help practitioners locate and utilise evidence so that they can produce personalised strategies for improving health and well-being that respond to local conditions and circumstances. The final section, Person Centred Approaches to Planning, will explore how evidence might be adapted to address the specific needs of individuals with learning disabilities.

ENHANCING SAFETY, COMFORT AND UNDERSTANDING

Northway et al. (2006) have suggested that inclusive and collaborative approaches are an intrinsic part of any solution that is likely to overcome persistent barriers to social inclusion. Actions that have been taken to enhance access to mainstream health services for people with learning disabilities include measures to facilitate the exchange of knowledge and experience between members of the extended healthcare team. Humber Mental Health Teaching NHS Trust et al. (n.d.) have developed a patient passport that arrives with a person with learning disabilities when they enter a service where he or she is not known. The patient passport document should be completed before a person enters a service by people who know the individual very well so that it is an accurate representation of their strengths, needs, likes and dislikes. It has been created so that staff providing care in the new setting will have the information necessary to enable them to develop a detailed picture of the individual's needs and to encourage them to work with that individual so that he or she feels safer, more comfortable and better understood.

Summarising basic information about an individual and conveying it to staff at the point at which the individual will receive a service might help to alleviate some of the problems that have been associated with the feelings of disorientation that can overpower people with learning disabilities when they enter an unfamiliar environment. Bollands and Jones (2002) have stated that the sort of information that a passport contains would be difficult to acquire by staff using the standard information gathering tools that are available in a hospital setting. Atkinson et al. have recognised that people with learning disabilities are likely to experience high levels of anxiety when they are confronted with a strange environment and this is most likely to be reduced when healthcare professionals work together to improve communication and 'the manipulation and coordination of the patient experience' (2010: 20). Passports might convey details about an individual's medical condition, religion, next of kin, personal care, communication, eating and drinking, likes, dislikes and advance decisions. Practitioners who possess this information can use it to anticipate or identify problems that they might de-escalate or avert so that an uncomfortable and unsettling episode is avoided.

The passport is not a universal plan; it is a template that can be used to collate and organise any information about an individual that has a direct bearing on their health and well-being. Iacono and David (cited in Backer et al., 2009) have identified a number of problems that people have encountered while they have been in hospital. These problems include getting to the toilet. Not everyone with a learning disability is going to experience a problem getting to the toilet, nor is there a simple correlation between the level of their impairments and the problems that they are likely to experience. A person with significant physical impairments who has the ability to make him or herself understood may experience fewer problems getting to the toilet than someone who is more mobile but cannot communicate. A person who cannot communicate effectively will find it difficult to make others aware of the sort of assistance that they need, and the communication gap is likely to be widest where the individual and the people providing care have no knowledge of one another. The passport can be used to convey information about how an individual prefers to use the toilet and other things that staff need to know about the ways in which an individual manages their continence or incontinence. For example, details might include the following:

How an individual makes a carer aware that he/she needs to use the toilet:

- whether the person can use single words e.g. 'toilet', or constructs sentences
- if the person does not communicate verbally, the passport might describe behaviours that indicate specific needs, for example noises or actions that may become more frequent and urgent if the individual feels that they are likely to wet and/or soil him/herself.

How much support an individual will need to get to the toilet:

- how far he/she can walk without assistance?
- whether he/she needs rails or other adaptations to enable him/her to use the toilet.

Routines:

- whether he or she is likely to be constipated
- what he or she does or takes to encourage a bowel motion.

Aids:

- the type/style/make of continence product that the person prefers.

Iacono and David (cited in Backer et al., 2009) and Fox and Wilson (cited in Backer et al., 2009) have also identified a number of issues relating to food and drink. The issues that they have mentioned include getting enough to drink and making choices from menus. To improve the experience of a person with learning disabilities in hospital a passport might contain the following:

Details about a person's personal preferences:

- likes and dislikes may include the meals an individual prefers to eat (or to avoid), specific tastes, textures, presentation and colours, as well as allergies.

How an individual makes another person aware that he/she is hungry or thirsty:

- by using words, pointing to pictures or using gestures
- how a person might indicate that he/she is not hungry now but would like to eat something later.

How much assistance a person needs with eating and drinking:

- whether the person needs help with the whole task
- whether the person can do some of the task by him/herself, for example can transfer a loaded spoon to his/her mouth but requires assistance to cut food into pieces of an edible size and cannot load them on a spoon/fork independently.

Whether an individual requires any special implements to help them to eat independently:

- whether a person needs a cup/beaker with one handle (or two) and/or a lid to drink independently
- whether a person requires a bowl or plate with a flattened lip (to push food against) to load a fork or spoon independently
- whether a person requires cutlery with built-up handles and grips to manage knives, forks and spoons independently.

EVIDENCE RELATED TO HEALTH INEQUALITIES

Practitioners who work with people with learning disabilities will need to be able to make use of different sorts of information. They will need to be able to translate detailed personal information, like the information that is recorded in a passport, into plans of care that reflect or are suited to the individual characteristics of the person receiving care. While practitioners should retain the principles of person centred practice and resist templates or stereotypes that do not recognise individual differences, they should not overlook information which is useful in conveying the bigger picture. Information in this category might look at national or international data relating to people with learning disabilities. Health inequalities are a way of examining the differences that influence the health of different populations or groups within a population. Differences can be the result of a combination of:

- biological factors – hereditary and genetic factors, factors related to age and gender
- social factors – lifestyle, housing, employment

- healthcare – access to health treatment
- health promotion – the impact of screening and the early detection of health problems.

Information on health inequalities can be an amalgamation of evidence from a range of different sources. It is often used to direct and focus health policy and practice. The Cabinet Office Social Exclusion Task Force (2010) produced an evidence pack which contains material related to socially excluded groups that include people with learning disabilities. The document has identified health risks and social determinants and provided examples of each (see Tables 8.1 and 8.2).

TABLE 8.1   *Evidence – The Cabinet Office Social Exclusion Task Force*

Health risks	Evidence – The Cabinet Office Social Exclusion Task Force
Mental health	Mental health problems are more common among adults with learning disabilities – prevalence of schizophrenia is around three times greater than for the general population
	27% of respondents to the Adults with Learning Difficulties survey reported experiencing mental health problems
Osteoporosis	People with a learning disability tend to have osteoporosis younger than the general population and to have more fractures
Respiratory disease	Three times more likely to die from respiratory disease
Heart problems	Higher risk of coronary heart disease than the general population and is the second most common cause of death in people with learning disabilities
Physical disability	Up to a third of people with learning disabilities have an associated physical disability
Weight	People with learning disabilities are more likely to be over or underweight e.g. 32% of women with LD are obese, compared with 23% of women in general population and 19% of men with learning disabilities were underweight compared with 2% of men in the general population

(Evidence from the Cabinet Office Social Exclusion Task Force 2010: 51)

The Department of Health Commissioning and System Management Directorate (2009) have compiled a similar list of health inequalities that has incorporated references to the research by Hollins et al. (1998). As well as referring to the health risks that are included in the Social Exclusion Task Force document this list also refers to:

- Forty per cent of people with learning disabilities have a hearing impairment and many have common visual impairments
- the rate of dementia is four times higher and the rate of schizophrenia three times higher than in the general population

- epilepsy is over 20 times more common in people with learning disabilities than in the general population. Sudden unexplained death in epilepsy is five times more common in people with learning disabilities than in others with epilepsy. (DH Commissioning and System Management, 2009: 15)

TABLE 8.2   *Evidence – The Cabinet Office Social Exclusion Task Force*

Social determinant	Evidence
Poverty	Severe learning disability is relatively evenly spread in the population. However mild to moderate learning disability rates are higher in some deprived and urban areas
	People with learning disabilities living in private households are much more likely to live in areas characterised by high levels of social deprivation
Income and employment	The employment rate among those in receipt of adult social services is just 10% – although 65% of people with learning disabilities would like to get a paid job
	Just 17% of people with mild/moderate learning disabilities and 4% of people with severe learning disabilities who were of working age reported earning more than £100 a week
Education and skills	Just over one in three people were undertaking some form of education or training. This was much higher among people with mild/moderate learning disabilities and severe learning disabilities than those with profound and multiple learning disabilities
Housing	The majority of people with learning disabilities, both mild and severe, live with a parent. People with more severe learning disabilities are more likely to be living in residential care homes and NHS accommodation
Lifestyle and behaviours	30% of those with mild/moderate learning disabilities reported smoking; 11% of those with severe learning disabilities and 4% of those with profound and multiple learning disabilities

(Evidence from the Cabinet Office Social Exclusion Task Force 2010: 51)

Mansell (2010: 24) has also identified some additional risks facing people with profound intellectual and multiple disabilities. These are:

- postural care: failing to protect body shape, damaging movement breathing and eating
- dysphagia: problems swallowing, damaging nutrition, breathing and resistance to infection
- pain and distress: failing to provide effective pain relief and treatment for the underlying cause.

Healthcare for All (Michael Report, 2008) indentified a range of factors that have contributed to the health inequalities experienced by people with learning disabilities. It included the findings from Hollins et al. (1998) which suggested that people with learning disabilities are 58 times more likely to die before the age of 50 than the rest of the population. In addition to the health problems that have already been identified there is additional evidence which showed that people with learning disabilities have had problems getting access to the resources that are needed to improve their health. When they are compared with the rest of the population, people with learning disabilities have fewer measurements of their BMI, those that have had strokes have fewer blood pressure checks, and cervical screening and mammography are less likely to be offered (Michael Report, 2008: 17). Early identification of problems can stop some preventable conditions from developing and allow more effective management of long-term health problems but for some people with learning disabilities the early detection and treatment of health problems has been impeded by diagnostic overshadowing. The Michael Report (2008: 18) refers to the Disability Rights Commission's (2006: 69) description of diagnostic overshadowing which states that it is a tendency to attribute symptoms and behaviour that are part of an illness to an individual's learning disability. The Disability Rights Commission (2006: 69) also reported that when some people with learning disabilities and their families told health professionals about changes in their physical health they were explained as 'behavioural'; this had meant that their experience of pain or a significant physical illness had been overlooked.

The Michael Report (2008) has identified a number of problems related to communication. Some people with learning disabilities find it difficult to express their needs to healthcare practitioners, for example they may find it hard to describe symptoms of an illness to another person. Some people may find it difficult to understand the information that they need to navigate healthcare systems, for example the process for referrals and appointments or understanding the differences between general and specialised services. Some people with learning disabilities find it hard to make their needs known because health professionals do not appear to want to listen to them (Michael Report, 2008: 16). Parents and carers of adults and children with learning disabilities also experienced this problem. Although they provide a significant proportion of care they are not seen as credible partners by professionals, even when they offer detailed knowledge and demonstrate their understanding of the people that they support.

The main body of the Michael Report (2008) contained ten recommendations for improving healthcare. The recommendations advised the

Department of Health to ensure that PCTs secured general health services that made reasonable adjustments to include people with learning disabilities. Adjustments should show compliance with, and enforcement of, the Disability Discrimination Act (2005) and the Mental Capacity Act (2005). In addition to ensuring compliance with these Acts the recommendations stated that the Department of Health should direct PCTs to commission enhanced primary care services that incorporated regular health checks by GPs, improvements in data collection related to the health and well-being of people with learning disabilities, better communication and cross-boundary working. Cross-boundary working should involve liaison with staff from different services to improve the health of people with learning disabilities across the spectrum of care. There were also specific recommendations that addressed the need to make improvements in undergraduate and postgraduate training. The recommendations stated that people with learning disabilities should be involved in training activities for practitioners. There was also a recommendation that practitioners should regard family carers (and other carers) as partners unless there were good reasons for not doing so. Partnership entailed the production of information in a format that they could understand as well as practical support and coordinating services.

Becoming familiar with the range of literature on health inequalities and being aware of the recommendations contained in the Michael Report (2008) are steps towards developing evidence based practice. To continue to develop the process practitioners are encouraged to combine the findings from research and other sources of literature with other sources of evidence. When a range of evidence has been identified, practitioners can develop specific plans and strategies that will enable them to adapt or apply evidence to meet the individual needs of clients or patients with learning disabilities. The next section in this chapter looks at models that incorporate different sources of evidence and how they might inform a practitioner's judgement. The final section describes some of the principles consistent with person centred approaches to planning. This section will also include case studies which provide you with an opportunity to identify goals that might improve the health and well-being of two fictional characters.

EVIDENCE BASED PRACTICE

Burton and Chapman (2004) have suggested that the relationship between theory and practice has acquired an orthodoxy that can deter practitioners from developing an effective evidence base. They have stated that the realities of complex service provision in the community, and particularly the 'complex and multifactoral nature of making interventions in health and social care' (Burton and Chapman, 2004: 59) make it difficult to produce scientific evidence that appears to address real life situations and problems. To encourage the development of stronger links between theory and practice they have described two models; one that looked at the sources of theory (Figure 8.1) and another that looked at different levels of evidence (Figure 8.2). The first model involved assembling a range of materials from different sources that will enable practitioners to develop a deeper understanding of a particular topic or situation. The materials used at this stage included formal studies derived from scientific research and literature as well as knowledge derived from first-hand experience, other people's experience and reflection.

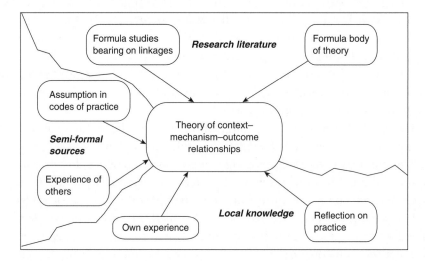

FIGURE 8.1   *Theory and Context–Mechanism–Outcomes Relationships*

The second model involved appraising the evidence and making decisions about its value in practice. The decision-making process considered evidence on three levels: macro, meso and micro.

Macro level evidence included research from primary and secondary sources, for example research articles, systematic reviews, and national guidelines. Meso level evidence incorporated material from established services or a population in a specific locality, for example audits, surveys, censuses of the local population. Micro level evidence included information related to specific individuals or groups, for example information from family members about an individual's behaviour or illness.

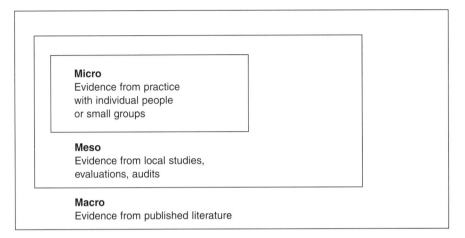

Micro
Evidence from practice
with individual people
or small groups

Meso
Evidence from local studies,
evaluations, audits

Macro
Evidence from published literature

FIGURE 8.2   *Levels to Consider in Decision Making*

The different stages in each of the models give practitioners an opportunity to evaluate evidence from different sources and to consider the advantages and disadvantages of applying it from the client's perspective. These processes may seem long-winded but they lend themselves to developing person centred strategies and encourage practitioners to move beyond the sort of orthodox thinking which can become fixated on methodological purity without applying the same rigour to translating and applying the findings so that they lead to practical solutions. Mantzoukas (2007) has also suggested that it is important to combine an understanding of the production of primary and secondary sources of evidence with the capacity to reflect on their usefulness. Reflection affords practitioners further opportunities to revisit their previous experience (including any knowledge they have acquired relating to specific clients or families) and to contemplate their own strengths and weaknesses. This will put them in a good position to think about whether they have the aptitude, skills and/or resources to initiate some strategies, whether they need to devote time and resources to acquiring them before they start, or whether they need to seek additional input from other teams/practitioners.

PERSON CENTRED APPROACHES TO PLANNING

Preparation and planning at the micro level entails gathering the sort of information that will help practitioners to form a better impression of the client's view of the world. This sort of information might record how an individual expresses themselves, for example his or her ability to convey thoughts and ideas through language, whether the individual makes regular use of signs or symbols, whether they use specific behaviours that communicate intentions or feelings. It might also record the most effective methods for communicating with that individual, for example language enhanced with photographs that function as objects of reference. Information will come from clients and carers and it will guide the development of strategies that enable clients to participate in the process. To ensure that the plan is realistic and that it addresses the day-to-day life of an individual it should also incorporate some contextual information which describes that individual's environment and the impact that it is likely to have on him/her. This type of information might refer to family or social networks, the resources that are accessible in the local community or the problems associated with gaining access to them. A person centred approach will mean that people with learning disabilities will have opportunities to benefit from practitioners' specialised knowledge but they should not be put in a position where they always need to defer to the practitioner's authority.

Nurses and other healthcare practitioners have developed specialised knowledge about health but to utilise that knowledge in a manner that is consistent with a person centred approach they must establish a shared understanding which allows them to work with clients as partners. In addition to the listening skills that are required to gather accurate information from clients, carers and family members, practitioners must also find ways of translating and conveying complex information about health so that it is accessible to people with learning disabilities. Read through the following scenarios that describe two people with learning disabilities.

Scenario

Jaid Singh is a 40-year-old man living in central Manchester. He is a sociable man with good communication skills. He is capable of understanding written information when it is produced in plain English. Jaid lives in shared accommodation with another man and a woman. They do not require a lot of support from staff but Jaid has sought some advice about his diet because he has noticed that he keeps putting on weight and he does not like it. He has a BMI of 29. He enjoys cooking and shopping with his housemates. He is not a fussy eater and he really likes his food. Jaid likes to visit the local shops and will purchase snacks during the day; sugary drinks and crisps are his favourites. He likes watching sport on television and going through his collection of films on DVD. He has expressed an interest in going out more and getting regular exercise but he has not committed himself to a specific activity.

Scenario

Miriam Lodge is a 35 year old woman who lives on the outskirts of Edinburgh. She lives with her parents. She has an older brother and a sister and the whole family are in regular contact although her brother and sister have their own homes and families. Miriam has cerebral palsy and epilepsy and uses a wheelchair. She does not speak but she can use vocalisations, gestures and facial expressions to convey her likes and dislikes. She is putting on weight because she loves eating and her parents encourage her to enjoy her food. Hilary and John (Miriam's parents) have said that eating is something that they can all enjoy together and because Miriam does not get out much they think giving her the sort of food that she likes is a way of improving the quality of her life. Miriam really enjoys chips, pies, cakes and pastries. She enjoys all sorts of food and does not reject anything in particular, but her preference is for sweet things. Miriam has a BMI of 27.

A person centred plan for Jaid or Miriam will bring together different types of evidence from a range of sources, that is material from macro, meso and micro levels.

Macro level evidence

You might start a search for evidence with an electronic literature search to locate material on health and well-being. The search could incorporate some databases that contain health-related research (e.g. CINAHL, BNI, MEDLINE) and some that are focussed specifically on people with learning disabilities (e.g. http://www.library.nhs.uk/learningdisabilities/). You might also include specific publications that address topics like healthy eating and/or obesity, for example the resources available from NHS Evidence/ National Library of Guidelines such as SIGN (2010).

Reflection Point 22

Think about how you might find specific information related to people with learning disabilities and how you might translate this information into material that is comprehensible to Jaid and Miriam. Make notes about the sort of goals that might appear in a care plan and who might be involved in helping the characters to achieve them.

(Continued)

Then note the search terms you might use to initiate an electronic literature search that would produce research relevant to Jaid and Miriam. Think about the differences that would result from using terms like 'healthy lifestyles', or 'healthy eating' and 'diabetes' or 'obesity', or 'obesity and people with learning disabilities'.

What might a search tell you about the risks that Jaid and Miriam are likely to face later in their lives if they continue to put on weight during their 30s and 40s?

Meso level evidence

Additional evidence might be gathered from specific health profiles relating to a district or county, for example Jaid and Miriam live in cities so practitioners in that area will refer to material that is available from the relevant Public Health Observatory (2010).

Evidence should also incorporate material about the services that are available in the locality. These might include:

- information about local health services, for example NHS Lothian (2010)
- information about specialised health services/practitioners, for example Manchester CLDT (n.d.)
- information about private, statutory, voluntary and charitable organisations in the area – material might address sport, leisure/recreation as well as health services, for example the resources that are available from Edinburgh City Council (n.d.)
- information about support/advocacy groups, for example, the resources available from Bristol and South Gloucestershire People First (n.d).

Reflection Point 23

Add some detail to the work from Reflection Point 22, show what you think about:

The range of services, organisations and practitioners that might be useful to Jaid and Miriam.

The contributions of 'generic' and 'specialised' practitioners. Does either character need a specialised service? Why? Might that character require a learning disabilities 'specialist' or another type of specialist, for example a dietician, an educator?

Access to the generic services/resources in your area. If you do think that Jaid/Mariam might find access to a particular service difficult, then identify the difficulties and make some suggestions for improving access. Start by thinking about the problems and then some solutions. Problems may be due to language, the process of making appointments, understanding the role of different practitioners, understanding the concepts that underpin healthy eating, a balanced diet, etc.

Micro level evidence

Evidence at this level will be gathered from Jaid, Miriam and/or their carers.

Reflection Point 24

Continuing from Reflection Point 23, add some detail to show what you think about:

The most effective ways of making Jaid, Miriam and/or their carers conscious of the risks that they may face in the future.

Ways in which you might adapt or supplement information so that it is suited to the individual needs of Jaid, Miriam and/or their carers. How would you present information, for example discussion, leaflets, text, pictures, DVDs?

A process for working with Jaid/Miriam and carers so that a practitioner will be able to negotiate goals or outcomes and gain consent to proceed with a plan. Do you present information so clients and carers can 'take it or leave it' or do you think about strategies for developing a more sustainable relationship? If you are considering a longer-term working relationship, how might you establish a rapport and develop trust with Jaid or Miriam? (For guidance see: *Valuing People Now* (2010))

Figure 8.3 from the Department of Health (2010) shows a range of outcomes that need to be achieved to deliver an effective person centered plan.

Specialist learning disabilities practitioners may contribute to health plans in different ways. They may be involved in one-to-one work with a person with learning disabilities that will result in the production of a plan that captures his or her individual needs and preferences. They may also work with people with learning disabilities, carers and health professionals who are based in primary or secondary healthcare services to assist with the production and implementation of plans. In this instance the plan might be used to communicate the needs and preferences of an individual with learning disabilities to professionals who do not know the person and/or professionals who have infrequent contact with people with

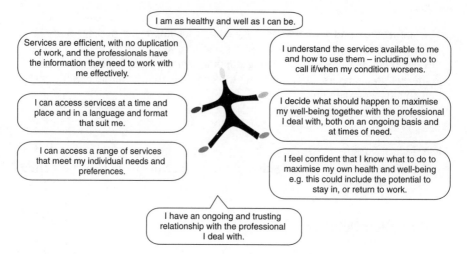

FIGURE 8.3   *Required Outcomes of an Effective Person Centred Plan (DH, 2010: 8)*

learning disabilities. The aim is to produce a document that will prepare local health services so that they can respond in a positive way to an individual's needs. Developing effective working relationships with people with learning disabilities and carers is a pivotal task for health professionals. An effective working relationship will promote trust and encourage the exchange of information about any decisions and choices connected with an individual's health and well-being. The implementation of a plan is likely to involve practitioners from other disciplines as well as those with experience and knowledge of learning disabilities, so practitioners deployed across the full range of health services might cultivate the values, skills and knowledge that will enable them to communicate successfully with people with learning disabilities and their families.

CONCLUSION

The content of this chapter has outlined some of the ways in which different practitioners can contribute to the development of an effective plan. For an individual with learning disabilities or a family carer to be able to make informed decisions about healthcare, they will need accurate and up-to-date information about risks and the range of treatments. This material may be derived from resources that are accessible to healthcare practitioners, for example specialised databases, journals, as well as practitioner based evidence and knowledge from those close to the person and from the person themself. People with learning disabilities will also need to have accurate and realistic advice on the range of services that are available in their locality. To make the most effective use of this information it will need to be presented to people with learning disabilities and carers so that they can understand it and discuss it prior to making any decisions about the care they want and/or need. This has repercussions relating to the type of materials that are best for the person, for example the combination of text, images, words that an individual is most likely to comprehend, as well as the amount of time that is required to prepare materials, clients and families so that they can use any information they receive to inform their decision making.

REFERENCES

Atkinson, D., Boulter, P., Pointu, A., Thomas, B. and Moulster, G. (2010) 'Learning disability nursing: how to refocus the profession', *Learning Disability Practice*, 13 (1): 18–21.

Backer, C., Chapman, M. and Mitchell, D. (2009) 'Access to secondary healthcare for people with intellectual disabilities: a review of the literature', *Journal of Applied Research in Intellectual Disabilities*, 22: 514–25.

Bollands, R. and Jones, A. (2002) 'Improving care for people with learning disabilities', *Nursing Times*, 98: 38–9.

Bristol and South Gloucestershire People First (n.d.) [online]. Available from http://www.bsgpf.org.uk/, accessed 27.06.2011.

Burton, M. and Chapman, M. (2004) 'Problems of evidence based practice in community based services', *Journal of Learning Disabilities*, 8 (56): 56–70.

Cabinet Office Social Exclusion Task Force (2010) *Inclusion Health Evidence Pack*. London: Department of Health. [online] Available from: http://www.cabinetoffice. gov.uk/social_exclusion_task_force/short_studies/health-care.aspxom, accessed 02.05.2010.

Department of Health (2001) *Valuing People: A New Strategy for Learning Disability for the 21st Century*. London: Department of Health.

Department of Health Commissioning and System Management Directorate (2009) *Improving the Health and Well-being of People with Learning Disabilities*. London: Department of Health.

Department of Health (2010) *Improving the Health and Well-being of People with Long Term Conditions*. [online] Available from: http://www.dh.gov.uk/en/Publicationsandstatistics/ Publications/PublicationsPolicyAndGuidance/DH_111122, accessed 02.05.2010.

Disability Discrimination Act (2005) London: HMSO.

Disability Rights Commission (2006) *Equal Treatment: Closing the Gap. A Formal Investigation into Physical Health Inequalities Experienced by People with Learning Disabilities and/or Mental Health Problems*. [online] Available from: http://83.137.212.42/

sitearchive/DRC/library/health_investigation.html#Finalreportsandsummaries, accessed 02.03.10.

Edinburgh City Council (n.d.) Home Page [website] Available from http://www.edinburgh.gov.uk/, accessed 06.04.2011.

Hollins, S., Attard, M.T., von Fraunhofer, N., McGuigan, S. and Sedgewick, P. (1998) 'Mortality in people with learning disability: risks, causes and death certification findings in London', *Developmental and Child Neurology*, 40: 127–32.

Humber Mental Health Teaching NHS Trust, Hull and East Yorkshire Hospitals NHS Trust, NHS East Riding of Yorkshire, NHS Hull (n.d.) *Patient Passport*. [online] Available from http://www.hey.nhs.uk/userfiles/file/patientpassport.pdf, accessed 06.04.2011.

Manchester CLDT (n.d) Home Page [website] Available from http://www.mldp.org.uk/cldt.htm, accessed 06.04.2011.

Mansell, J. (2010) *Raising our Sights: Services for Adults with Profound Intellectual and Multiple Disabilities* [online] Available from: http://www.dh.gov.uk/en/Publicationsandstatistics/Publications/PublicationsPolicyAndGuidance/DH_114346, accessed 02.05.2010.

Mantzoukas, S. (2007) 'A review of evidence-based practice, nursing research and reflection: levelling the hierarchy', *Journal of Clinical Nursing*, 17: 214–23.

Mental Capacity Act (2005) London: HMSO.

Michael Report (2008) *Healthcare For All: Report of the Independent Inquiry into Access to Healthcare for People with Learning Disabilities*. London: Department of Health.

NHS Lothian (2010) Home Page [online] Available from http://www.nhslothian.scot.nhs.uk/, accessed 06.04.2011.

Northway, R., Hutchinson, C. and Kingdom, A. (2006) *Shaping the Future: A Vision for Learning Disability Nursing*. London: UK Learning Disability Consultant Network.

Nursing and Midwifery Council (NMC) (2008) *The Code: standards of conduct, performance and ethics for nurses and midwives*. [online] Available from: http://www.nmc-uk.org/Nurses-and-midwives/The-code/The-code-in-full/, accessed 26.03.2011.

Public Health Observatory (2010) 'New health profiles for every local authority in England', *Health Profiles*. [online] Available from: http://www.improvinghealthandlives.org.uk/, accessed 20.04.2010.

SIGN (2010) *Management of Obesity*. Edinburgh: Scottish Intercollegiate Guidelines Network. [online] Available from: http://www.sign.ac.uk/guidelines/fulltext/115/index.html, accessed 20.04.2010.

Valuing People Now (2010) *Healthy Lives Project*. [online] Available from: http://valuingpeople.gov.uk/dynamic/valuingpeople143.jsp, accessed 20.04.2010.

9

EPILEPSY, PAIN AND END OF LIFE CARE: HEALTHCARE ISSUES FOR PEOPLE WITH LEARNING DISABILITIES

Amelia Oughtibridge

INTRODUCTION

This chapter will focus on some common health issues that affect people with learning disabilities. Mansell, in his report on services for people with profound and multiple learning disabilities, made specific recommendations about healthcare, stating that:

> NHS bodies should ensure they provide health services to adults with profound intellectual and multiple disabilities in each area which focus on protection of body shape, dysphagia, epilepsy and investigation and resolution of pain and distress. (2010: 24)

Where the NHS works to improve service for this most vulnerable group the learning and expertise that develops will have positive impacts for all people with learning disabilities. Caring for a person who has intractable epilepsy, managing someone who is unable to verbalise their pain, and caring for someone with a learning disability who is at the end of their life can be challenging to many health professionals. Therefore, this chapter seeks to use these examples of health needs to draw together what makes people with learning disabilities so complex and how to ensure best healthcare.

HEALTH ASSESSMENT

The most important factor when working with people with learning disabilities is to be prepared for communication difficulties. Because it can be difficult to communicate, one can assume that the person cannot understand or offer any reliable information for the assessment. Never make assumptions about what the person with learning disabilities can or cannot understand; however, assessment starts with some fundamental reasoning:

- the likely underlying physical cause for the presenting symptoms/problems will need perseverance to establish
- the presenting symptoms are likely to have more than one causal factor.

People with learning disabilities will require more time to be included in their own healthcare to aid understanding. Health services are required to make reasonable adjustments to ensure services are accessible to people with learning disabilities (Michael Report, 2008). Affording extra time is the most cost-effective adjustment services can offer people with learning disabilities within mainstream health services. A common cause of poor healthcare for people with learning disabilities is a lack of understanding and skill in assessment. This can be for a myriad of reasons, one of which is confidence. Nurses and doctors will often say, 'I have had no training in caring for people with learning disabilities', believing that specialist services have the expertise. However, specialist services cannot replace primary, secondary or dental services and people working in mainstream services often forget the transferable skills they have.

Differential diagnosis refers to an assessment process when we need to understand a health problem for which there are multiple symptoms, possible causes and environmental factors at play and is used in situations where individuals cannot tell you about their illness or how they are feeling. In such circumstances, assessments based on obtaining a detailed patient history and accounts of the symptoms are the norm. The practitioner forms an hypothesis using their clinical reasoning, available evidence and clinical experience alongside appropriate test results combined with the patient's accounts of their illness. This leads to a diagnosis. However, for people who are unable to communicate this information the health professional will need to rely on an assessment that involves carer observation and knowledge of the patient as well as the usual forms of evidence. It is essential that the practitioner guard against diagnostic overshadowing when making any diagnosis (see Chapter 8 for a definition of diagnostic overshadowing).

Assessment for people with learning disabilities should cover all the aspects one would cover for anyone else, but with due consideration to the following:

- History
- Mental capacity
- Vulnerability
- A final point here is also to establish what is usual good health for this patient – a base line, that indicates what best health looks like for this person.

History

People commonly present with a myriad of problems, resulting in a confusing picture. A health history and family history are important parts of any initial assessment. This can be difficult to obtain from someone who uses non-verbal communication or does not know the language to use. The nature of learning disability can lead a person to have difficulty relating to time; they may tell you about something in the present tense but it may have happened some time ago or vice versa.

The residential environments people live in can result in carers who may know the person well but have inaccurate information, especially about history. Support workers and family members who know the person well should be included in supporting the assessment but not to the exclusion of the person themselves or without their consent. It can be useful to develop a background history including information from the person's GP. In England GPs are involved in a Direct Enhanced Service (DES), providing annual health checks for people with learning disabilities (NHS, 2008a). The health check ensures people's health needs are met at primary care level and provide a record of underlying conditions such as diabetes or hypothyroidism. A general health check is often the best place to start for most problems. It will rule out possible conditions contributing to the presenting issue, such as hypothyroidism, helicobacter pylori and anaemia. There is no doubt that annual health checks for people with learning disabilities provide health gains (Felce et al., 2008).

Consent and Mental Capacity

It is the responsibility of every health professional to gain consent for treatment and to assess the person's ability to be involved in their own healthcare (DH, 2001). Many people with learning disabilities will need either support for this or require the multi-disciplinary team to make decisions in their best interests. However, health professionals, hospitals and doctors frighten some people with learning disabilities and others will not be able to tolerate a procedure such as a blood test, a dental examination or invasive procedure such as cervical cytology. Where this is the case, it is important that the reason for the suggested test is documented. It is not appropriate to take 'no further action' without a sound rationale. Careful consideration is needed as to why the person cannot tolerate the procedure and if there is anything that could be done to support the person to overcome their fears (DH, 2001). Giving information in a way that makes sense to the person can often overcome fears and misunderstandings the person holds (see www.easyhealth.org.uk for examples of accessible health information).

Assumptions about capacity to consent are illegal and often lead to poor health outcomes for people with learning disabilities. The Mental Capacity Act (2005) supports decision making and practitioners should always use the best interest pathway to document the outcome of decisions. Following careful consideration of capacity, if the procedure is essential and in the person's best interest, plans to support the person to have the procedure are recorded. The scenario below is an example of how thorough assessment helped Janet have good healthcare.

Scenario

During the annual health check, the GP noticed Janet was showing symptoms of lethargy, dry skin, and weight gain. The GP wanted to offer Janet a blood test to find out if she had hypothyroidism. The GP's assessment of Janet was that she lacked capacity to consent to the blood test. However, she continued with her assessment of Janet to see if Janet would be able to have the test with minimum distress. She checked with Janet's family if she had tolerated blood tests previously. Her mother said that Janet could have blood taken if people were prepared to sing songs with Janet, while a skilled phlebotomist carried out the procedure. The GP also asked how Janet would show distress, which was recorded by the GP. The GP explained the need for the blood test and the possible health gains for Janet to the family, who agreed the test would be in Janet's best interests. They planned to use Janet's love of singing and music to distract her, but agreed to stop at any point if Janet showed signs of distress. The specialist nurses showed how to hold Janet's arm safely for the procedure. Janet had the blood test at the surgery and showed no signs of distress. She flinched when the needle went in her arm but the supporting nurse was able to hold her arm gently. With everyone, including Janet, singing away to Abba songs the blood test was carried out.

Janet needed treatment for an underactive thyroid. The correct dose was iden-tified for Janet with subsequent blood tests and her health improved. The GP used assessment skills tailored to her patient's needs and applied reasonable adjustments to the service she provided.

Vulnerability and Risk

People with learning disabilities are extremely vulnerable in hospital (Mencap, 2007). Some hospitals have learning disabilities liaison nurses who assist with specialist expertise; others link with learning disability teams to support hospital admission and discharge. Specialist support establishes exactly what is available to make the experience safe for the person as well as adding value to the health outcomes for the individual.

Reflection Point 25

Do you have access to a hospital liaison nurse either in your own NHS Trust or through a Community Learning Disabilities Team? If you do, what is their role and how would you contact them if you had someone with a learning disability admitted for treatment where you work?

Vulnerability increases through complexity; for example where the person's health is affected by long-term conditions that are often associated and co-exist with the learning disability, such as physical or sensory impairments, epilepsy, mental illness or dementia. Where the person has a profound learning disability the possibility of having sensory and physical impairment and epilepsy is much higher (Pawlyn and Carnaby, 2009). Multiple carers, multiple or temporary care environments or sudden changes in psychosocial circumstances – such as loss and bereavement – add to this complexity. Combined with communication difficulties a picture of complexity that often requires specialist assessment and intervention develops (Mencap, 2001). Therefore, it is important that you identify additional risk factors so you can put support in place to effectively and safely manage associated risks.

It has been documented that people with learning disabilities have suffered from preventable deaths and co-morbidity due to healthcare that does not work for them (Disability Rights Commission, 2006; Emerson and Baines, 2010). Through examining the person's risk factors at initial assessment you will be able to ensure that the risks are known and documented and managed to lessen the risk.

EPILEPSY

Approximately 30 per cent of people with learning disabilities have epilepsy with the incidence rising to 50 per cent of people with severe learning disabilities (Foundation for People with Learning Disabilities, 2002). This is due to the underlying brain damage that results in both the learning disability and a higher risk of epilepsy. It is easy to have low expectations of seizure control in people with learning disabilities because of the high incidence but this should be challenged.

Specialists, often within multi-professional teams, care for people with learning disabilities with complex epilepsy (NICE, 2004a). This is because control can be very difficult to achieve due to the complexity of diagnosis and continued treatment. Poor control is often due to the aetiology of the brain, but can be compounded by extreme sensitivity to medication and environmental factors. Poor practice in epilepsy care is a contributor to poor control, the effects of which the individual has to live with every day. Kerr et al. (2009) highlight the issues regarding treating people with learning disabilities who have epilepsy. There is high incidence of poly-pharmacology (more than one anti-epileptic medication) and poor quality medication reviews that encompass diagnostic overshadowing. Often people will present with partial seizures (where the seizure activity is happening in a focal part of the brain and, therefore, the person may be conscious or partially conscious and behaving strangely) that are mistaken for behavioural problems (NICE, 2004a). Conversely, there is a high risk of diagnosing epilepsy when the seizures are actually not epilepsy. Kerr et al. (2009) have produced guidelines that relate to identifying epilepsy and seizure patterns in this population with particular emphasis on the reporting of what happened before, during and following the seizure incident. This report must be as accurate as possible and NICE (2004a) suggest a video of the incidents as most reliable. Recording is important as the frequency, length and timing of the seizures can support diagnosis, continued care, treatment and medication variations. The National Society for Epilepsy has information about the types of seizures and further information about epilepsy (www.epilepsysociety.org.uk/Homepage).

When caring for someone with learning disabilities who has epilepsy there are common features to include in assessment. Considering the person's epilepsy is important, regardless of whether your involvement is directly associated with the person's epilepsy. In all healthcare environments, regular seizure activity must be quickly identified and treated as it is a serious medical issue. It is important to identify the person's seizure pattern and plan what to do if they have a seizure while in your care. Carers can be a useful resource when understanding a person's epilepsy. If seizure activity is suspected make a note of the following:

- What is observed: a description of what the seizure looks like, how long it lasts and recovery.
- Treatment: what medication do they take, in what form and what is the dose? What non-pharmaceutical treatment do they have?
- What does best care look like if the person has a seizure? Do they have any rescue medication? If so, when should it be given?

Recording the answers to these questions or obtaining a copy of the person's epilepsy care plan will enable you to provide continuing care throughout an admission to an acute hospital department. Some people will have frequent seizures that are difficult to control and can be subject to changing patterns. It is critical that any changes in usual seizure activity are taken seriously and treated appropriately. Seizure changes might require further examination and review of current treatment. It is always worth considering if modern examinations could benefit the ongoing assessment and care of the individual. As assessment and treatment in epilepsy care advances (such as MRI scans) it is possible for improved care. Through lowering the seizure frequency or severity we can improve not only individual's quality of life but also increase life expectancy. Sudden Unexplained Death in Epilepsy (SUDEP) is a known cause of death in people with epilepsy. Although we are not fully aware of the mechanisms that cause SUDEP, seizure control can reduce the risk (NICE, 2004a).

Status Epilepticus

For the patient who has 'hard to treat' epilepsy (Kerr et al., 2009) there will be a higher risk of prolonged seizures (Status Epilepticus). Rescue medication (Buccal Midazolam or rectal Diazepam) is prescribed to stop prolonged seizure activity, or clusters of seizures (NICE, 2004b). Individuals will have a care plan for when their rescue medication is given. Buccal Midazolam is now more popular because it is less invasive, however, the person administering it must have received training in its safe use (NICE, 2004b).

PAIN

'Pain is what the patient says it is and exists whenever he or she says it does' (McCaffery and Beebe, 1999). This holistic definition referred to pain that might be caused by emotional or spiritual distress as well as physical pain and is useful because it reminds us that the experience of pain is subjective to the patient. However, exercise caution in the application of this definition for people with learning disabilities because of the reliance on patient self-description of what they are feeling. The emphasis is on the communication of pain descriptors such as burning, tingling, radiating, and sore pressure or stabbing. Someone might open up about a loved one or a memory that could be the cause of their anguish. They often need to be able to say where they feel the pain and when they feel it. Some health professionals use pain assessment tools – for example pictures of smiley faces with expressions of pain – to support the pain assessment. However, for some people with learning disabilities, pain might not be describable as individuals might not know the language of pain and its complex descriptors. The more severe the learning disability the more difficult it will be for the person to describe or alert people to their pain. Pain is therefore one of the most commonly overlooked areas of healthcare for people with learning disabilities, often left untreated or under treated (Kerr and Wilkinson, 2006).

Very often people with learning disabilities express pain through body language or unusual expressions, for example laughter. This is often coupled with assumptions, myths and false beliefs about people with learning disabilities including notions that they cannot feel pain or have a 'high pain threshold'. This is a myth that holds no place in the healthcare of people with learning disabilities. There is no doubt that people have suffered as a result of these myths and assumptions (Kerr and Wilkinson, 2006). In their study on pain and dementia in people with learning disabilities, Kerr and Wilkinson (2006) found that pain was not recognised and noted that symptoms such as night waking were not attributed to pain. They related their findings to older people generally and found that people with learning disabilities were less likely to receive treatment for painful conditions such as arthritis. In discussing pain recognition, Kerr and Wilkinson (2006) found that people who challenged with behavioural difficulties were not treated for pain. In many circumstances, the behaviour was attributed to the learning disability (diagnostic overshadowing). Health professionals have a duty to recognise pain in this patient group and to enable the people close to them to understand how pain can be communicated and recognised in someone who cannot verbally communicate. Assessment involves understanding what a person's pain or distress signals will look like, knowing what they are likely to be and then observing for them.

The *DisDAT* tool (Northumberland Tyne and Wear NHS Trust and St. Oswald's Hospice, 2008) is a distress assessment tool that highlights in detail the person's behaviours and signals when they are not in distress, which form a base line. Once this is in place, a record of what distress looks like for the person is recorded offering health carers something to observe for, report and react to. The tool is effective in helping to recognise pain in people with idiosyncratic communication skills (Regnard et al., 2007). The next step is to work out using differential diagnosis assessment what could be causing the distress and how to alleviate it.

Reflection Point 26

Think of someone you have supported who may not have been able to tell about their pain.

What body language, facial expressions and sounds might have indicated pain in your patient?

How could you record these idiosyncratic ways of demonstrating pain so others could identify their pain?

Pain management with analgesia

It is important to apply good practice for pain management to people with learning disabilities. WHO (1996) advises considering the following five points when treating cancer pain:

- by mouth
- by the clock
- by the ladder
- attention to the individual
- attention to detail.

When working with people with learning disabilities, following these principles will enable the consideration of providing treatment in a person centred way. This increases the chance of treatment having positive outcomes for the patient who is experiencing pain. This is especially useful if you are treating someone who lacks capacity and for whom you are considering treatment in their best interests and we recommend this model for using analgesia for any pain or distress.

By Mouth

Considering medication given by mouth should be the first line approach of treatment. Through considering the least invasive medication you will promote independence and dignity for the person. If medication is to be administered by an alternative route provide evidence why this is required. Person centred approaches to care are fundamental to good practice, as in the following example.

Scenario

Sandra is a woman with learning disabilities who has a diagnosis of lung cancer. She has autism and people who do not know her very well find communicating with her very difficult. However, her family and carers are saying that she is in more pain and discomfort and needs something to treat her pain. Although normally she loves going out with her family lately she remains in her room. Her interest in food has also deteriorated.

Sandra will not take tablets or liquid medication; she has spat them out in the past. She does not understand that the tablets could help her to feel better. The nurse explains that there is a patch available that sticks on the skin, but it can take three days for the medication to get into the system. A problem can be that the amount of medication in the system cannot be as easily changed as it can with oral medication. During a meeting with the nurse and GP it was agreed with the family that treatment with the patch was in Sandra's best interests. They would start with the lowest dose patch and monitor over the next three days. The carer would put the patch on Sandra after her bath. A record was kept of how and where the patch was put on. Carers monitored for any change in Sandra during the following days and nights. Gradually Sandra improved and came out of her room; she even wanted something to eat. The patch was continued and was an effective pain treatment for Sandra.

By the Clock

A basic principal of pain relief is for medication to be given at regular intervals. The dose should be in line with being effective in relieving the pain. The intervals should be in time to prevent the pain breaking through. It is important that this basic rule is followed for people with learning disabilities to enable the effectiveness of the medication. The person themselves should be as independent as possible and involved in their own care. Some useful pictorial information is available to support individuals to self-medicate (see CHANGE, n.d.). However, you can draw a clock to explain the importance of how to gain effective relief from pain. A dosette box or an alarm watch can increase effective regular self-administration of medication and should be considered to promote independence. If the person with learning disabilities relies on carers, the emphasis is on their education.

Carers have a significant role to play in the effective treatment of pain for people with learning disabilities. Carers can sometimes hold their own beliefs about medication or perhaps worry that they are over medicating the person they care for. Paid carers as well as family carers will need information to enhance their understanding, especially if opioids are prescribed. Check they know what the medication is for, how it works and its benefits. Make sure they know that the medication is to control symptoms and is not curative.

There should be regular reviews and reassurance that the medication is still needed because carers sometimes feel that because a person is symptom free, they no longer need medication. Help them to know what the common side effects are and think about what signs are likely to be observable.

By the ladder

WHO (1996) outline using the least powerful medication initially and titrating up to more powerful drugs according to the degree of pain control gained. This is well known by health professionals and is of benefit for the following reasons:

- The principals of the ladder are easily understood by carers and will increase their confidence in your practice. Tell them the approach you are taking, tell them about the medications used at each level and where on the ladder the individual is
- The ladder can support a systematic approach that will ensure effective relief of symptoms with the right drug at the right time
- The approach will ensure the right drug is targeting the right symptom, for example when treating different types of pain
- This approach is in line with the principals of differential diagnosis by following a process of elimination of symptoms alongside effectiveness of the medication.

Attention to the individual

Pain management is based on what the person says about their pain (WHO, 1996). This means that medication, its dose and effectiveness, is based on the individual and not on universal guidance. It is important to gain good quality information to inform practice so getting to know the person with learning disabilities is particularly important when applying this principle. Individuals and carers should keep a pain diary to enable 24-hour monitoring of pain and distress. Such a diary can show patterns in the presentation of the symptoms and support a diagnosis or hypothesis. Use language that everyone understands rather than the medical terms or usual descriptors of pain.

Scenario

Janet's diary records her distress throughout the day. We know that if she cries out loud, it means she is uncomfortable and wants someone or something, for example she might do this because she might want to be moved or is hungry. This does not happen often because she is cheerful and her carers anticipate her needs. However, if she cries silently it means pain that relates to her arthritis. We know this because she cried silently a lot before she was treated for pain. On having treatment, her silent crying lessened. Janet's pain diary started to show an increase in silent crying again. It showed her distress regularly appeared an hour before the next dose of her medication. Her nurse interpreted it as break-through pain. Following careful alteration of Janet's medication her silent crying reduced again.

People who knew Janet helped the health professionals involved in Janet's care to understand her individual communication of her pain. Always try to achieve consensus of what the person is communicating because there are often subtle differences (Regnard et al., 2007).

Attention to detail

This final but most critical aspect of care cannot be emphasised enough when assessing and treating people with learning disabilities for pain. It could be through giving more time, analysis of diaries and understanding complex communication. Such detail could result in health intervention making a real difference. Here is an account of Danielle who was discharged from hospital to her flat after being diagnosed with terminal cancer.

Scenario

Danielle did not like being in hospital and once she got home would ask her carers if she would have to go back saying she did not want to go back to hospital. The district nurse wanted to find out what Danielle understood about her diagnosis. The notes from the hospital showed that staff had discussed her diagnosis with her and there were some hand drawn pictures showing where the cancer was. The nurse showed the pictures to Danielle and she became extremely upset, shouted no and wanted the nurse to leave. The next time the nurse visited, she came in normal clothes. She had reflected on the previous visit with a colleague and they wondered if Danielle's reaction was because she thought she had to go to hospital. Danielle seemed more at ease with the nurse. The nurse reassured Danielle that she did not have to return to hospital and that they could help her to stay in her flat. After some weeks of visiting in normal clothes, the nurse was able to use the pictures again with Danielle. Subsequently they used them to pinpoint and manage her pain.

The attention to detail and adjustments that this nurse made resulted in her forming a good relationship with Danielle. She understood that Danielle was trying to communicate and she took a different approach to establish another way of supporting her.

END OF LIFE CARE

The End of Life Care Strategy (DH, 2008) guides us towards good practice in end of life care. The publication of the *Routes to Success in End of Life Care* (NHS, 2011a) further promotes the needs of people with learning disabilities. It outlines best practice and seeks to involve the patient and their family, offering the help and support to enable people to die with dignity. There are various tools to support practice, such as *Advanced Care Planning* (NHS, 2008b) and the Liverpool Care Pathway (Ellershaw and Wilkinson, 2010). *The National End of Life Care Programme* (NHS, 2011a) has published practical guidance based on six steps that will enable a team to provide care based on compassion and quality (NHS, 2011b).

The principle of partnership, working with the team of people who are around the individual, is core to best practice in achieving the best outcomes for the individual. Most people want a good death by having a life right up until death, to feel that staff know what they are doing and that they are not a burden on them, having freedom from pain and other distressing symptoms, while knowing that loved ones are cared for. The team of people aiming for this should be whoever it needs to be, with an open and transparent system for knowing the role and responsibility of everyone in the support team. The team is likely to be made up of professionals from palliative care services, primary GP services and specialist learning disability services working together to coordinate advanced care planning through linking end of life care with the individual's person centred plan (NHS, 2011a). Family and paid carers are likely to play a large part and it is important to get the balance right for them in terms of their caring role. Paid support carers in learning disabilities services will form a significant part of the social and spiritual care for the person, as well as being in a prime position to monitor for signs of symptoms and distress because they know the person so well. However, an over reliance on these carers can lead to disastrous results for them and the individual.

Scenario

Stewart lived in a residential care home for people with learning disabilities. He loved his mother and his sister who visited most days and he often went out with them. He loved the outdoors, to feel the wind in his face. The diagnosis of advanced cancer was a shock for everyone. Stewart did not have the capacity to understand his diagnosis and was therefore dependent on his carers in the home and his family to anticipate his needs. The care home staff decided they would care for Stewart in the home, but they did not realise just how ill he would become. They did not have any experience of terminal illness and were not used to providing intensive physical care for their residents. They were not aware of what was likely to happen or given any information about the disease trajectory. They found it very painful indeed to see him become thin and could not cope with the extra care they needed to give him. They felt overwhelmed and worried that Stewart was in pain and they did not know what to do about it.

Reflection Point 27

Left to continue, this situation would break down and the result will be very poor experiences for Stewart and his family. How could the team support Stewart and his carers?

The principle of partnership can help you to resolve some of the issues we have seen in Stewart's case. What can you reasonably expect informal carers and paid carers to do for someone in their care who is dying?

What can you do to make sure that Stewart is not at risk from unrecognised or undertreated symptoms?

Mainstream health services play a pivotal role in the care of someone who is dying and supporting social care staff and family towards offering the care that they feel competent and confident to give, and no more. Healthcare staff need to identify carers' levels of confidence and competence and offer appropriate support sharing what they know about end of life care and ill health (NHS, 2011b). Specialist staff can establish if carers have the skills, resources, knowledge and understanding to care for the person in the family home, their own home or a residential home. Good partnership working will enable the identification of what care the person will need from services. The responsibility of meeting the needs of the person who is dying lies with health staff and not with the social care team or the family. Stewart was in danger of poor care because of an over reliance on the care home to meet all of his needs.

Scenario

Following on with Stewart.   The district nursing team recognised the complexity of Stewart's care. They met with the local hospice team and GP to discuss the way forward. They clinically assessed Stewart and worked with the homecare staff and the family. Concerned that they could not assess Stewart properly, the palliative care nurse arranged for Stewart to stay at the hospice for a few days. He took his health action plan and communication plan with him so the hospice staff could learn how to communicate with him. He benefited from consistency in care and his family had an opportunity to talk and use the hospice services. Stewart stabilised and returned to his home with a detailed end of life care plan.

Meanwhile the home staff had an opportunity to reflect on the care they could give to Stewart and his family, and were supported by the learning disability nurse and district nurse to consider their role. They realised that they were not alone and other services would help. They used person centred thinking tools developed by Kennedy, Broadley and Helen Sanderson Associates (2008) to help them understand Stewart's changing needs and how they could help him. They balanced this with what was important for Stewart and identified how they could make sure he got the best care balanced with experiences he loved. This meant that before he died Stewart did some lovely things with this friends and family, supported by the care staff. Partnership working ensured he got a wheelchair when required, his symptoms were well controlled and the hospice staff came in which helped the care staff to have breaks and spend time with the other residents. Stewart died peacefully in his home. The hospice and district nurses followed up with bereavement care.

Stewart's example shows how mainstream health services and professionals can use their expertise leading on the principle of partnership. Health staff have expertise and access to advanced skills that ensure positive outcomes in end of life care.

CONCLUSION

It is common to hear health professionals say that they cannot work well with people with learning disabilities because of a lack of training and experience. This chapter has aimed to give some ideas about how everyone can get involved in the assessment and treatment of people with learning disabilities. Advancing skills and confidence in the workforce of professionals associated with healthcare will bring about transformation for people with learning disabilities. Knowledge of the common health inequalities, health problems and issues that can create barriers to good health for this population will open up mainstream practice towards excellence.

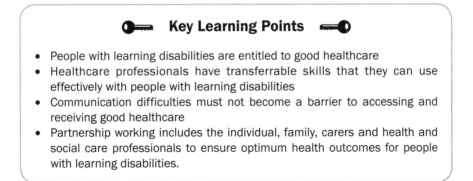

🔑 Key Learning Points 🔑

- People with learning disabilities are entitled to good healthcare
- Healthcare professionals have transferrable skills that they can use effectively with people with learning disabilities
- Communication difficulties must not become a barrier to accessing and receiving good healthcare
- Partnership working includes the individual, family, carers and health and social care professionals to ensure optimum health outcomes for people with learning disabilities.

REFERENCES

CHANGE (n.d.) *Health Picture Bank.* [online] Available from http://www.change-people.co.uk/pictureBank.php?id=1722, accessed 23.11.2010.

Department of Health (2001) *Seeking Consent:Working with People with Learning Disabilities.* [online] Available from http://www.dh.gov.uk/en/Publicationsandstatistics/Publications/PublicationsPolicyAndGuidance/DH_4007861, accessed 19.03.2011.

Department of Health (2008) *The End of Life Care Strategy.* London: Department of Health.

Disability Rights Commission (DRC) (2006) *Equal Treatment – Closing the Gap.* Stratford Upon Avon: Disability Rights Commission.

Ellershaw, J. and Wilkinson, S. (2010) *Care of the Dying: A Pathway to Excellence* (2nd edn). Oxford: Oxford University Press.

Emerson, E. and Baines, S. (2010) *Health Inequalities and People with Learning Disabilities in the UK: 2010.* Improving Health and Lives. London: Learning Disability Observatory and NHS.

Felce, D., Baxter, H., Lowe, K., Dunstan, F., Houston, H., Jones, G., Felce, J. and Kerr, M. (2008) 'The impact of repeated health checks for adults with intellectual disabilities', *Journal of Applied Research in Intellectual Disabilities*, 2: 585–96.

Foundation for People with Learning Disabilities (2002) *Epilepsy and Learning Disabilities.* [online] Available from http://www.learningdisabilities.org.uk/information/syndromes-and-conditions/epilepsy/?locale=en, accessed 23.11.2010.

Kennedy, S., Broadley, J. and Helen Sanderson Associates (2008) *Person Centred Thinking and Health.* [online] Available from http://www.hsapress.co.uk/publications/mini-books.aspx, accessed 19.03.2011.

Kerr, D. and Wilkinson, H. (2006) 'Responding to the pain needs of people with a learning disability/intellectual disability and dementia: what are the key lessons?', *International Journal on Disability and Human Development Special Issue*, 5 (1): 69–75.

Kerr, M., Scheepers. M., Arvio, M., Beavis, J., Brandt, C., Brown, S., Huber, B., Livanainen, M., Louisse, A., Martin, P., Marson, A., Prasher, V., Singh, B., Veendrick, M. and Wallace, R. (2009) 'Consensus guidelines into the management of epilepsy in adults with an intellectual disability', *Journal of Intellectual Disability Research*, 53 (8): 687–94.

Mansell, J. (2010) *Raising Our Sights: Services for Adults with Profound Intellectual and Multiple Disabilities.* London: Department of Health.

McCaffery, M. and Beebe, A. (1999) *Pain: Clinical Manual for Nursing Practice* (2nd edn). St Louis: Mosby.

Mencap (2001) *No Ordinary Life.* London: Mencap.

Mencap (2007) *Death by Indifference.* London: Mencap.

Mental Capacity Act (2005). London: HMSO.

Michael Report (2008) *Healthcare for All: Report of the Independent Inquiry into Access to Healthcare for People with Learning Disabilities.* [on-line] Available from http://www.dh.gov.uk/en/Publicationsandstatistics/Publications/PublicationsPolicyAndGuidance/DH_099255, accessed 19.9.2009.

National Health Service (2008a) *Primary Care Contracting: Primary Medical Care New Clinical DES /Summary for PCTs / PCC / PMC / GMS.* [online] Available from http://www.pcc.nhs.uk/uploads/primary_medical/new_clinical__des_summary_for_pcts__pcc_pmc_gms_guidance_web_cd__23_09_08.pdf, accessed 12.12.2008.

National Health Service (2008b) *Advanced Care Planning: A Guide for Health and Social Care Staff.* [online] Available from http://www.endoflifecareforadults.nhs.uk/publications/pubacpguide, accessed 19.03.2011.

National Health Service (2011a) *National End Of Life Care Programme: The Route to Success in End of Life Care – Achieving Quality for People with Learning Disabilities.* [online] Available from http://www.endoflifecareforadults.nhs.uk/publications/route-to-success-people-with-learning-disabilities, accessed 19.03.2011.

National Health Service (2011b) *National End of Life Care Plan.* [online] Available from http://www.endoflifecareforadults.nhs.uk/care-pathway/1-initial-discussion, accessed 19.3.2011.

National Institute for Clinical Excellence (NICE) (2004a) *The Epilepsies: The Diagnosis and Management of the Epilepsies in Adults and Children in Primary and Secondary Care.* London: National Institute for Clinical Excellence.

National Institute for Clinical Excellence (2004b) *Quick Reference Guide. The Epilepsies: Diagnosis and Management of the Epilepsies in Children and Young People in Primary and Secondary Care.* London: National Institute for Clinical Excellence.

Northumberland Tyne and Wear NHS Trust and St. Oswald's Hospice (2008) *DisDAT.* [online] Available from http://www.crfr.ac.uk/disdat/Assess%20tool%2009.pdf, accessed 21.11.2010.

Pawlyn, J. and Carnaby, S. (eds) (2009) *Profound Intellectual and Multiple Disabilities: Nursing Complex Needs.* Oxford: Wiley-Blackwell.

Regnard, C., Reynolds, J., Watson, B., Matthews, D., Gibson, L. and Clarke, C. (2007) 'Understanding distress in people with severe communication difficulties: developing and assessing the Disability Distress Assessment Tool (DisDAT)', *Journal of Intellectual Disability Research,* 51(4): 277–92.

World Health Organisation (WHO) (1996) *Cancer Pain Relief* (2nd edn). [online] Available from http://whqlibdoc.who.int/publications/9241544821.pdf, accessed 23.11.2010.

10 MEETING SOME SPECIFIC MENTAL HEALTH NEEDS OF PEOPLE WITH LEARNING DISABILITIES

Alan Nuttall

INTRODUCTION

The study of mental ill health in people with learning disabilities is still a relatively new field. Even twenty years ago, it was generally felt that people with learning disabilities did not experience mental ill health and there was no significant body of literature or research relating to this topic. Neither were members of the nursing branch for this specialised client group given much training in the manifestation and treatment of psychiatric illness (Lindsey, 2003), even though they were often supporting people in a nominally hospital setting, under the auspices of psychiatric consultants. Although the psychiatric consultant was often referred to as being 'the responsible medical officer', his or her role was predominantly administrative, rather than medical.

In recent times research has established that people with learning disabilities are possibly up to three times more likely to develop mental illness than the general population (Moss and Lee, 2001). Partly this is because there are several conditions such as autism, Fragile X and Down's syndrome among others associated with learning disabilities, which predispose to psychiatric disorders like anxiety or dementia. Also, this group are more prone to be subjected to certain psychological and social vulnerability factors for emotional disorders. For example, they are more likely to endure separation and loss, struggle to develop supportive networks of friends, be subjected to changes and life events beyond their control, suffer all forms of abuse including sexual and physical abuse, and be disadvantaged financially (Bailey and Jackson, 2003).

This chapter will explore some of these vulnerability issues and will discuss difficulties with diagnosis and assessment. A range of treatments and interventions, including the uses of and warnings against psychotropic medication and psychological treatments, will be highlighted. Two examples of mental ill health in people with learning disabilities are also offered in this chapter. First, alcohol and drug abuse – often attributed to an increased exposure to community facilities and the risk of exploitation – is examined. Second dementia is highlighted, specifically exploring the correlation between Alzheimer's disease in Down's syndrome. The chapter concludes with a brief commentary on mental health law including the Mental Capacity Act (2005) and tensions that exist between specialist learning disability services and generic mental health services for people with learning disabilities and additional mental health needs.

DIAGNOSIS AND ASSESSMENT

Diagnosis of psychiatric disorder in people with learning disabilities can be difficult. Signs and symptoms as presented by adults with mild learning disabilities and reasonable communication skills may well be similar, albeit in a less complex manifestation, to those exhibited by the general population. However, it is likely that people with a severe disability or autism may display disturbed or dysfunctional behaviour or else display physical ill health as possible indicators of poor mental health (Gravestock et al., 2005). Challenging behaviour, defined classically by Emerson as:

> culturally abnormal behaviour of such intensity, frequency or duration that the physical safety of the person or others is likely to be placed in severe jeopardy, or behaviour which is likely to seriously limit or deny access to and the use of ordinary community facilities. (1995, cited in Emerson, 2001: 3)

is the most likely reason for a referral to a specialist psychiatric consultant. However, although a part of the ICD 10 and DC-LD diagnostic classification systems (Royal College of Psychiatrists, 2001), challenging behaviour is not a clinical diagnosis in itself and can often be explained by environmental factors such as noise, overcrowding, boredom, or inability effectively to communicate needs or pain and discomfort, rather than psychiatric disorder (Clarke, 2006).

Frequently clinicians can interpret phenomena as being an intrinsic aspect of a person's disability when they are in fact indicative of psychiatric disorder, a well-documented process known as diagnostic overshadowing (Mason and Scior, 2004). Conversely, over diagnosis may occur because the disorganised thoughts, behaviour and speech of someone of a limited developmental ability are interpreted as signs of psychosis.

Hardy and Bouras (2002) suggest many strategies to overcome difficulties in diagnosing and assessing the mental state of people with intellectual disabilities. These include seeing the person in their natural environment. If this is not possible then make sure that the individual is fully orientated to the clinical environment prior to attending for assessment. It is important that any communication difficulties or sensory deficits are acknowledged and compensated for. The environment should be comfortable, free of distractions and predictable. Open-ended questions and simple, concrete terminology should be used, while reference to events such as Christmas or birthdays can be used if the person being assessed has difficulties with times and dates. Individuals should be supported by someone who knows them really well and information from those who knew the individual before symptoms became apparent is valuable.

Several tools have now been developed either to assess mental ill health or alert carers of its possible onset. An example of the former is the Psychiatric Assessment Schedule for Adults with a Developmental Disability (PAS-ADD) interview while the PAS-ADD Checklist has been established by Sturmey et al. (2005) as a reliable screening tool for use by support staff. Prosser et al. (1998) confirm the reliability and validity of the Mini PAS-ADD and assert it is a suitable tool for non psychiatrists and an effective link between the expertise of psychiatrists and psychologists and the knowledge of clients possessed by support workers. Other assessment formats are the Learning Disability version of the Cardinal Needs Schedule (Raghavan et al., 2004) and the Diagnostic Assessment for the Severely Handicapped–II (DASH-II) described by Bamburg et al., (2001).

Scenario

Linda was born into a poor family in a deprived area of a large city. It was apparent from an early age that she had a mild learning disability.

Her father left the family home when she was four years old, never to return or re-establish any contact. Linda's mother married again and had more children, her family eventually numbering six. However, Linda's step-father, whom she liked, died before she became a teenager. Her mother then developed a relationship with a man who repeatedly sexually abused Linda and punished her in humiliating ways. Subsequently, Linda started displaying unusual behaviour, including exposing herself through her bedroom window and being aggressive to others. She started attending a 'special school', which involved lengthy travelling each day, and was bullied and teased.

When she left school, she became involved in a relationship with a man who often used her as a prostitute or took and sold her possessions. She left the family home and lived in at least twenty locations over the next four years, including a squat, hostels, foster homes, care homes and NHS treatment units, pursuing a chaotic and promiscuous lifestyle and being diagnosed at this point as having a personality disorder. She then moved to a newly opened care home where she lived for several years, for the first time having the support of a consistent team for a lengthy period of time. Although the team were inexperienced in the support of someone with Linda's complexities, they were able to arrive at an empathic understanding of her history and how it affected her behaviour and the way she lived her life. She continued to lead a wayward lifestyle, in which she was frequently sexually exploited by men and encouraged to take recreational drugs. She often became irritable and aggressive to others and started to complain of hearing voices. After an attack on her mother during a visit to her home, she was admitted to a Treatment and Assessment Centre and diagnosed as having paranoid schizophrenia. Her original staff team continued to stay in touch with Linda and, although she had a period of over a year living in several NHS settings, eventually she requested to return to the care home. By then she was receiving treatment appropriate to her illness and, although still occasionally having aggressive outbursts and putting herself in potentially abusive situations, began associating with a more supportive peer group and acting more responsibly. Thirteen years after her initial move to the care home she was able to move into her own flat.

Linda's history shows her exposure to different vulnerability factors, such as being born into poverty, exposure to abuse and exploitation, in turn leading to low self-esteem, bereavement and other adverse life events. It also demonstrates the difficulties of diagnosis; how a chaotic lifestyle, challenging behaviour and lack of opportunity to observe over a significant period of time can lead to misdiagnosis and inappropriate treatment. With regard to the staff team, it was many years before they gained a full appreciation of the nature and impact of Linda's mental illness, highlighting the need for training of carers in the presentation and assessment of psychiatric disorder.

> **Reflection Point 28**
>
> Think about the things that you have in your life that help you maintain your mental well-being. What supports do you have in your life that people with a learning disability might not have? Think about those people with learning disabilities who live independently as well as those living with family members or in a communal care environment.

TREATMENTS AND INTERVENTIONS

Psychotropic medication, developed and prescribed specifically for psychiatric disorders, is often the first recourse for treatment of apparent mental illness in people with learning disabilities. However, it is evident that a higher proportion of this group compared to the general population receive such medication, sometimes at higher doses than are recommended by the British National Formulary, the accepted guide in this matter (Deb, 2006).

Also, Chapman et al. (2006) identified that often psychotropic medication is prescribed when there is no clear diagnosis. Polypharmacy, that is the administration of several forms of medication, whether from the same category (for example more than one antipsychotic medication) or from several categories (for example antipsychotic drugs plus an antidepressant) often takes place.

A common reason for prescription of psychotropic drugs is the manifestation of disruptive behaviour, which may be a psychiatric phenomenon but could easily be due to lack of stimulation, inability to communicate needs effectively, a chaotic or noisy environment, or even physical ill health. Often those so treated remain on psychotropic medication for many years because of the perceived intractability of their behaviours, giving rise to increased liability to the development of neuroleptic malignant syndrome – a condition in which individuals display persistent unwanted side effects such as muscle rigidity or uncontrollable body movements similar to Parkinson's disease (Jenkins, 2000). Nevertheless, Clarke (2006) asserts that it is beyond reasonable doubt that psychotropic medication is effective in treating severe psychiatric disorders in all client groups, including the learning disabled, and Jenkins (2000) cautions against the denial of treatment with these types of drugs because the prevailing culture may be strongly against a medical approach to care.

Stenfert-Kroese et al. (2001) recommend that people prescribed psychotropic medication should be reviewed regularly by the multi-disciplinary team, should have a functional analysis of behaviours and symptoms prior to treatment to assess the impact of personal and environmental factors, and that such medication should never be used as a form of chemical restraint. People should either receive full information concerning their treatment in an accessible form or, if the service user has limited comprehension and communication ability, an independent advocate should be engaged. Also staff should receive sufficient training, particularly in the use and side effects of drugs, so that they can effectively and assertively contribute to reviews. Jenkins (2000) adds that it is important to ensure that all are clear which precise symptoms or condition the medication is being prescribed for and there is a clear process for assessing whether the target symptoms have had a positive response to the medication. Jenkins (2000) also argues that drug treatments should always be accompanied by other interventions. Stenfert-Kroese et al. (2001) argue further that interventions which are not reliant on medication and have a good evidence base for effectiveness should be preferred. In the past, there was a view that people with learning disabilities were not appropriate recipients of psychotherapeutic strategies such as Cognitive Behaviour Therapy, a phenomenon referred to as 'Therapeutic Disdain' by Bender (1993: 8).

Oliver and Smith (2005) describe the most common psychological interventions currently used. These include the behavioural approach in which observations are made of behaviours and objectively analysed in order to understand what is perpetuating the behaviour or what the person is trying to communicate by it, in order to help the client develop more effective ways to express themselves and achieve their needs. Recent studies have noted the effectiveness of Cognitive Behaviour Therapy (CBT) in reducing the impact of the symptoms of schizophrenia in those with a mild intellectual disability (Haddock et al., 2004) and the synergistic effect of using CBT in concert with treatment with the drug clozapine, also prescribed for schizophrenia (Turkington et al., 2004). Cognitive Behavioural Therapy addresses the phenomenon in which emotional problems arise from negative thoughts and beliefs, by helping the service user develop more positive thoughts and beliefs. Haddock et al. (2004) detail how sessions of CBT can be adapted to the needs of people with learning disabilities through careful attention to length, location and structure of sessions, with emphasis on these being relatively short, taking place in the person's home, and the use of pictures and videotapes to supplement written material. Person Centred Therapy (PCT), in which the service user is regarded as the expert about himself, assumes that the person's emotional problems occur because their experiences have been discounted or denied by others. Because this is often the case with people with learning disabilities PCT is seen as being an effective approach for them.

All carers and health professionals have a role to play in helping service users to enhance the protective factors that aid prevention of the onset of mental ill health; these include ensuring adequate nutrition and exercise, prompt treatment for physical ill health, development of relationship networks and development of social skills, assertiveness and self-esteem (Hardy and Bouras, 2002).

EXAMPLES OF MENTAL ILL HEALTH IN PEOPLE WITH LEARNING DISABILITIES

Alcohol and Drug Abuse

Almost two decades ago Lindsay et al. (1991) identified that people moving from the insular environment of a long-stay hospital to urban communities might have a greater risk of developing alcoholism. They suggested factors such as previous limited opportunities to experience community life, the perception that going to the pub was an accepted part of living in a town and limited means to explore other leisure options. People who were brought up in residential hospitals and would have been denied extensive opportunities to meet people and socialise may regard drinking in a local as a highly valued activity and be drawn to excessive alcohol intake that way. McMurran and Lismore (1993) cited evidence from American studies that there was a disproportionately high incidence of alcohol-related arrests associated with people who had a learning disability. In their study, Taggart et al. (2006) established that alcohol was the main substance abused but at least a fifth of the group that they examined used a combination of illicit drugs such as cannabis and ecstasy or prescription medication. They found that the propensity for substance abuse was more prevalent in young males with a mild learning disability and mental health difficulties. There is a consensus that people with learning disabilities are less likely to drink and take drugs but, if they do, have a greater tendency to have serious problems with addiction. Taggart et al., taking into account the views of those who do misuse alcohol and drugs, describe their actions as 'self medicating against life's negative experiences' (2007: 360), particularly the distress caused by unpleasant life events such as bereavement or abuse by partners, and the sense of estrangement from their community, being lonely and having few friends. They report the ineffectiveness of mainstream services in helping the clients that they interviewed, who described their anxiety about sharing experiences in group work but felt they benefited from one-to-one work with an addiction counsellor.

Lindsay et al. (1991) developed a comprehensive assessment and treatment strategy for an Alcohol Education Service specifically for this client group, including a checklist which explored reasons for drinking and a questionnaire which asked clients to reflect on the situations when they were likely to consume alcohol. This stage of assessment was used to encourage service users to reflect on alternatives to drinking alcohol, symptoms that they experienced after excessive drinking and the development of knowledge about alcohol. Each person was encouraged to fill out a drinking diary prior to attending sessions at the service and were taken to a local pub to be assessed with regard to the way they used alcohol (for example, speed of drinking, social behaviour). Subsequent interventions consisted of discussion to allow individuals to develop their understanding of why people drink, what they can do to moderate their intake, what is a safe amount to drink, and what actually constitutes being an alcoholic. In a later article, Lindsay et al. (1992) talked about clients who drink to help forget their worries and the difficulties in fostering motivation to lower intake. They felt that it was unrealistic to expect people to give up going to the pub completely; it was better to teach reasonable behaviour related to alcohol consumption – 'the Art of Positive Drinking' (Lindsay et al., 1992: 46). Manhope (1997) asserts the importance of service providers ensuring that a strict ban on consuming alcohol is imposed on support workers while they are on duty to provide clear and unambiguous role modelling around responsible drinking.

Scenario

Arthur lived in long-stay institutions from the age of 13, moving twice from hospitals which were closing to other sites in the city that he lived. He was not considered to be someone who could readily settle into a community setting due to his complexities, which included autism, a dependence on the hospital culture and a history of being abused. During his last hospital placement, he became friendly with a group of people who frequented a local pub. They encouraged him to drink alcohol excessively and also to take drugs. He became neglectful of his personal care, sometimes verbally aggressive and stayed out late to the early hours of the morning, often coming back to the ward drunk or stoned, extremely unkempt and argumentative. Finally, while under the influence of alcohol and drugs he accidently cut his arm attempting to clear up some broken glass in the street. His refusal to allow treatment for what at the time was considered a potentially life threatening wound, involving nerve and ligament damage, led to his compulsory admission to a Treatment and Assessment Centre under a section of the Mental Health Act, where he received treatment for both

(Continued)

his physical and mental ill health. However, he could not return to his old hospital, the last remaining in the city, since it was only months from closure. Therefore, he was offered a place at a local care home which had gained a reputation for effective support of people with similar needs and lived there for eight years with some success and enjoyment, for the first time in his adult life having ready access to ordinary community facilities. However, throughout that time he constantly became involved with dysfunctional groups of people who encouraged him both to drink alcohol in excess and take illegal drugs, causing him to behave in a similar way to when he was living in his final hospital placement. With difficulty, it was possible to access treatment from the local alcohol rehabilitation service which was initially reasonably effective. It was clear though that practitioners in the alcohol rehabilitation service were unused to his particular client group. At times he was at risk from sexual exploitation and physical attack, on one occasion requiring hospital treatment for a head injury following a serious assault. Also his relationship with the local community deteriorated due to his argumentative, unkempt demeanour and inappropriate behaviour, such as openly urinating in neighbours' gardens. Finally, he moved to another home which had equally good community presence but was more secure, where it was possible both to help him moderate his alcohol intake and learn more appropriate rules of social behaviour.

Reflection Point 29

Read through the scenario above and list the things in Arthur's life that had made him susceptible to drug and alcohol abuse. What dilemmas do staff have to consider when supporting Arthur?

This scenario demonstrates the difficulties people who have lived the majority of their lives in an isolated setting may have in learning restraint in consuming alcohol or illicit drugs when exposed to normal community life, particularly if they are hampered in understanding social rules and norms due to autism. It shows the dilemmas between affording someone ready access to facilities and opportunities that had been denied them for most of their life and ensuring their protection from the dangers of alcoholism and recreational drug use. It also shows the need for alcohol rehabilitation services to be equipped to treat people with learning disabilities, and for staff to receive training in how to support and educate service users who abuse alcohol.

Dementia

The incidence of dementia in people with learning disabilities is generally the same as that experienced by the general population at about 5 per cent of those over the age of 65. The incidence for people with Down's syndrome is much higher, rising to over 50 per cent in the 60 plus age range. In this group dementia can occur as early as 40, the average age of onset being 54, with death often occurring within five years (Prasher, 1995). Consequently it is advised by Dodd et al. (2003) that people with Down's syndrome should be assessed at the age of 30 to establish a baseline of cognitive functioning and adaptive living skills in all settings that the person commonly experiences.

Many of the early signs of dementia – such as changes in mood, decline in daily living skills and disorientation – may be caused by environmental changes or other conditions like depression, thyroid problems and sensory impairment, all of which should be eliminated as possible causes or treated prior to a diagnosis of dementia (Turk and Dodd, 2005). Someone who knows the person well, including how they were in the more distant past, should always be present for information gathering interviews. Multiple assessments should take place, including assessment of medical history, past abilities, and the presence of possible risk factors like head injury or a family history of Alzheimer's disease. Psychosocial and psychiatric histories should encompass identifying any mental health problems, bereavements and significant life events that they might have experienced. There might be a need for hearing and sight tests, specific blood tests or CAT/MRI scans. Also cognitive and social abilities should be assessed as well as any tendency to behavioural changes (Turk and Dodd, 2005). The same writers assert the desirability of maintaining the person who has dementia in their own home as far as possible. If a move has to be made it should be to a setting which can accommodate the person as they subsequently deteriorate, to prevent further potentially disorientating moves. Alternatively adaptations should be made to the living environment as necessary to ensure that it remains suitable. It is essential for carers to be flexible and maintain a routine which is suited to the person with dementia rather than trying to impose a rigid routine. Increased supervision and prompting, keeping verbal communication simple, and the use of memory aids such as diaries, timetables and the compiling of a life history can all help the person maintain skills and compensate for memory loss. As dementia develops issues that might have to be addressed include agitation, hallucinations, delusions and the onset of epilepsy. In the later stages, physical health needs predominate as the person perhaps loses mobility, becomes prone to falls, develops the need for intensive skin care and may develop swallowing difficulties, necessitating involvement of such professionals as physiotherapists and speech therapists.

Scenario

Frances lived in a long stay hospital for most of her life and lost contact with her family. She had Down's syndrome, a condition which did not significantly impair her quality of life or ability to look after herself. When she was about 55 her paid carers noticed that she was starting to become restless at night, often walking around the home in the early hours of the morning. Usually cheery and sociable in manner, she increasingly seemed morose and introverted and gradually spoke less, to the point where she eventually did not speak at all. She lost the ability to dress and feed herself and also became incontinent. She also found walking more difficulty, developing stiffness in her gait until she lost that ability also. Towards the end of her life Frances started experiencing involuntary muscular spasms and also tonic-clonic epileptic seizures that required treatment by anticonvulsant medication. Throughout her decline the staff team had to adapt their approaches and care in a way which preserved Frances's dignity and sense of individuality when it was no longer possible to compensate for her deterioration.

Reflection Point 30

If you were looking after Frances what sort of augmentative communication systems might be in place to support Frances as her speech gradually declined? (See Table 7.1 for examples if needed.)

MENTAL HEALTH LAW

The Mental Health Act of 1983 set out provision for compulsory admission to hospital for assessment or treatment, either as an emergency for 72 hours (s. 4), assessment for 28 days (s. 2) or treatment for six months (s. 3) (Tewari, 2006). The most recent revision of Mental Health Law introduced the one term 'mental disorder', instead of the four terms used in the 1983 Act, which included mental impairment and severe mental impairment. Just having a learning disability should not be regarded as sufficient grounds for detention unless the learning disability is associated with 'abnormally aggressive or seriously irresponsible conduct' (Mental Health Act 2007: 2). Kramer (2007) feels that this is contrary to how the general population is treated, and will lead to many people with a learning disability remaining in hospital because of anti-social or criminal activity rather than mental illness. The 2007 Act also states that appropriate treatment must be available in the event of compulsory detention, which may not be the case in the above circumstances. Nevertheless, Kramer (2007) also states that given the propensity of people with an intellectual disability to be more susceptible to mental ill health than the rest of the population, it is important that the small minority of this group who need treatment under compulsory detention legislation have the same rights and safeguards appertaining to such treatment as anyone else. The Mental Health Act (2007) also introduced Deprivation of Liberty Safeguards to ensure the least restrictive care regimes for groups such as those with learning disabilities, dementia or mental ill health, and to prevent arbitrary and unlawful detention.

There are also provisions within the 2007 revision which allow for treatment within a community setting, either under Supervised Treatment, Supervised Discharge Orders, or Guardianship. The Act also states that a person discharged from hospital after a period of compulsory detention must be in receipt of a plan of care. Although not incorporated in the Act, the Care Programme Approach (CPA) has been developed for this purpose. CPA, with its emphasis on the primacy of the needs of the individual, a holistic approach and commitment to multi-disciplinary support, although not superseding a person centred plan can be seen as being compatible with the philosophy informing the latter.

The Mental Capacity Act of 2005 protects the rights of people with learning disabilities, irrespective of whether they also have a mental illness, by establishing that capacity to make decisions should be assumed unless there is compelling evidence to the contrary, that all practicable steps should be taken to help people make decisions rather than an assumption being made of an inability to do so, and that unwise decisions are not indicative of lack of capacity. There is provision to take decisions on behalf of those who do lack capacity, but only in their best interests and in the least restrictive way possible.

SPECIALIST SERVICES AND QUALITY ISSUES

Although *Valuing People* (DH, 2001) states that people with learning disabilities have a right to access general psychiatric services, mental health support is still usually provided by specialist teams. These Community Learning Disability Teams, consisting of many different professionals including social worker, specialist nurse, speech and language therapists, physiotherapists, clinical psychologist and consultant psychiatrist, have a wider focus than mental health alone and through pressure of referrals or insufficient training (for example, nurses may be trained only in the learning disabilities branch specialism) may not be the ideal way to support this group. However, these teams are repositories of knowledge concerning the specific needs of people with learning disabilities and can respond in a holistic way, maintaining people in their local communities through outpatient support, so preserving protective factors such as support from family and friends and continuity of interests and activities. Some areas have developed specialist mental health in learning disability services which are not necessarily a part of learning disability services and can facilitate treatment within mainstream adult psychiatric provision.

It is actually rare for people with intellectual disabilities to access mainstream mental health inpatient facilities, as staff feel ill-equipped to support this specialist group and there is a view that the general psychiatric environment is too frightening and volatile for this vulnerable client group (Vanstraelen et al., 2003). Therefore, inpatient treatment is usually provided by specialist treatment and assessment units. As well as NHS provision, a network of secure hospitals has come into being. Seen by some as asylums for people with troubled minds, usually these institutions are in remote locations which deny people their protective factors such as ready support of family and community presence, and by virtue of their potential insularity could easily perpetuate the abusive culture of the long-stay hospitals which were the main provision of care in the twentieth century.

Hall et al. (2006) describe a service in which mainstream mental health services work cooperatively with specialised learning disability practitioners to meet the needs of people with learning disabilities and mental ill health. Gibson (2009) reminds us that there are insufficient specialist services to deal with the volume of mental healthcare required in the intellectually disabled client group. Such services might not be available locally. Use of specialist services deny mainstream professionals the opportunity to develop skills in working with this group, while practitioners in general learning disability services may lack knowledge in mental health issues, making an integrated approach necessary in the future.

CONCLUSION

Considerable progress has been made over the last twenty years with regard to the understanding of the manifestation and effect of mental ill health on people with learning disabilities and the reasons for the greater incidence in this segment of the population. Methods of assessment have been developed which recognise the specific needs of this group and the range of treatments has been extended. Specialist services can give valuable support; however, it is important to develop such areas of expertise within generic services in line with modern approaches. The vast majority of people with learning disabilities now live in ordinary community settings; the challenge for the future is to ensure that professionals within all the services which they encounter are fully aware of the specific needs and supports that they require for effective prevention, diagnosis and treatment of mental ill health.

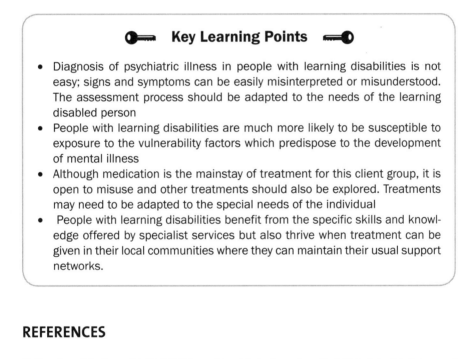

🔑 Key Learning Points 🔑

- Diagnosis of psychiatric illness in people with learning disabilities is not easy; signs and symptoms can be easily misinterpreted or misunderstood. The assessment process should be adapted to the needs of the learning disabled person
- People with learning disabilities are much more likely to be susceptible to exposure to the vulnerability factors which predispose to the development of mental illness
- Although medication is the mainstay of treatment for this client group, it is open to misuse and other treatments should also be explored. Treatments may need to be adapted to the special needs of the individual
- People with learning disabilities benefit from the specific skills and knowledge offered by specialist services but also thrive when treatment can be given in their local communities where they can maintain their usual support networks.

REFERENCES

Bailey, J. and Jackson, V. (2003) 'Mental health in learning disabilities', in M. Jukes and M. Bollard (2003) *Contemporary Learning Disability Practice*. Salisbury: Quay Books.

Bamburg, J.W., Cherry, K.E., Matson, J.L. and Penn, D. (2001) 'Assessment of schizophrenia in persons with severe and profound mental retardation using the Diagnostic assessment for the severely handicapped-11 (DASH-11)', *Journal of Developmental and Physical Disabilities*, 13 (4): 319–31.

Bender, M. (1993) 'The unoffered chair: the history of therapeutic disdain towards people with a learning disability', *Clinical Psychology Forum*, 54: 7–12.

Chapman, M., Gledhill, P., Jones, P., Burton, M. and Soni, S. (2006) 'The use of psychotropic medication with adults with learning disabilities: survey findings and implications for services', *British Journal of Learning Disabilities*, 34: 28–35.

Clarke, D. (2006) 'Psychiatric disorders and challenging behaviour', in A. Roy, M. Roy and D. Clarke (eds), *The Psychiatry of Intellectual Disability*. Oxford: Radcliffe Publishing.

Deb, S. (2006) 'The use of psychotropic drugs in people with intellectual disabilities', in A. Roy, M. Roy and D. Clarke (eds), *The Psychiatry of Intellectual Disability*. Oxford: Radcliffe Publishing.

Department of Health (2001) *Valuing People: A Strategy for People with Learning Disabilities in the 21st Century*. London: Department of Health.

Dodd, K., Turk, V. and Christmas, M. (2003) *Down's Syndrome and Dementia Resource Pack*. Kidderminster: British Institute of Learning Disabilities.

Emerson, E. (2001) *Challenging Behaviour: Analysis and Intervention in People with Learning Disabilities* (2nd edn). Cambridge: Cambridge University Press.

Gibson, T. (2009) 'People with learning disabilities in mental health settings', *Mental Health Practice*, 12 (7): 30–3.

Gravestock, S., Flynn, A. and Hemmings, C. (2005) 'Psychiatric disorders in adults with learning disabilities', in G. Holt, S. Hardy and N. Bouras (eds), *Mental Health in Learning Disabilities*. Brighton: Pavilion Press.

Haddock, G., Lobban, F., Hatton, C. and Carson, R. (2004) 'Cognitive-behaviour therapy for people with psychosis and mild intellectual disabilities: a case series', *Clinical Psychology and Psychotherapy*, 11: 282–98.

Hall, I., Parkes, C., Samuels, S. and Hassiots, A. (2006) 'Working across boundaries: clinical outcomes for an integrated mental health service for people with intellectual disabilities', *Journal of Intellectual Disability Research*, 50 (8): 598–607.

Hardy, S. and Bouras, N. (2002) 'The presentation and assessment of mental health problems in people with learning disabilities', *Learning Disability Practice*, 5 (3): 33–8.

Jenkins, R. (2000) 'Use of psychotropic medication in people with a learning disability', *British Journal of Nursing*, 9 (13): 844–50.

Kramer, R. (2007) 'The Mental Health Act for 2007: better or worse for people with learning disabilities?' *Learning Disability Today*, 7 (4):14.

Lindsay, W.R., Allen, R., Walker, P., Lawrenson, H. and Smith, A.H.W. (1991) 'An alcohol education service for people with learning disabilities', *Mental Handicap*, 19: 96–9.

Lindsay, W.R., Allen, R., Quinn, K., Walker, P. and Smith, A.H.W. (1992) 'The art of positive drinking', *Nursing Times*, 88 (25): 46–8.

Lindsey, M. (2003) 'New patterns of service', in W. Frazer and M. Kerr, (eds), *Seminars in the Psychiatry of Learning Disabilities* (2nd edn). London: Royal College of Psychiatrists.

Manhope, J. (1997) 'Service challenges: the pleasures and problems of alcohol', *Journal of Learning Disabilities for Nursing, Health and Social Care*, 1 (1): 31–6.

Mason, J. and Scior, K. (2004) '"Diagnostic overshadowing" amongst clinicians working with people with intellectual disabilities in the UK', *Journal of Applied Research in Intellectual Disabilities*, 17: 85–90.

McMurran, M. and Lismore, K. (1993) 'Using video tapes in alcohol interventions for people with learning disabilities. An exploratory study', *Mental Handicap*, 21: 29–31.

Mental Capacity Act (2005) London: HMSO.

Mental Health Act (1983) London: HMSO.

Mental Health Act (2007) London: HMSO.

Moss, S. and Lee, P. (2001) 'Mental health', in J. Thompson and S. Pickering (eds), *Meeting the Health Needs of People who have a Learning Disability*. London: Balliere Tindall.

Oliver, B. and Smith, P. (2005) 'Psychological interventions for people with learning disabilities', in G. Holt, S. Hardy and N. Bouras (eds), *Mental Health in Learning Disabilities*. Brighton: Pavilion Press.

Prasher, V. (1995) 'End-stage dementia in adults with Down's syndrome', *International Journal of Geriatric Psychiatry*, 10: 1067–9.

Prosser, H., Moss, S., Costello, H., Simpson, N., Patel, P. and Rowe, S. (1998) 'Reliability and validity of the Mini PAS-ADD for assessing psychiatric disorders in adults with intellectual disability', *Journal of Intellectual Disability Research*, 42 (4): 264–72.

Raghavan, R., Marshall, M., Lockwood, A. and Duggan, L. (2004) 'Assessing the needs of people with learning disabilities and mental illness: development of the Learning Disability version of the Cardinal Needs Schedule', *Journal of Intellectual Disability Research*, 48 (1): 25–36.

Royal College of Psychiatrists (2001) *Diagnostic Criteria for Psychiatric Disorders for Use with Adults with Learning Disabilities/ Mental Retardation (DC/LD)*. London: Gaskell Publishers.

Stenfert-Kroese, B., Dewhirst, D. and Holmes, G. (2001) 'Diagnosis and drugs: help or hindrance when people with learning disabilities have psychological problems', *British Journal of Learning Disabilities*, 29: 26–33.

Sturmey, P., Newton, J.T., Cowley, A., Bouras, N. and Holt, G. (2005) 'The PAS-ADD Checklist: independent replication of its psychometric properties in a community sample', *British Journal of Learning Disabilities*, 29: 319–23.

Taggart, L., McLaughlin, B., Quinn, B. and Milligan, V. (2006) 'An exploration of substance use in people with intellectual disabilities', *Journal of Intellectual Disability Research*, 50 (8): 588–97.

Taggart, L., McLaughlin, B., Quinn, B. and McFarlane, C. (2007) 'Listening to people with intellectual disabilities who misuse alcohol and drugs', *Health and Social Care in the Community*, 15 (4): 360–8.

Tewari, S. (2006) 'Intellectual disability and the law', in A. Roy, M. Roy and D. Clarke (eds), *The Psychiatry of Intellectual Disability*. Oxford: Radcliffe Publishing.

Turk, V. and Dodd, K. (2005) 'Mental health problems in older people with learning disabilities', in G. Holt, S. Hardy and N. Bouras (eds), *Mental Health in Learning Disabilities*. Brighton: Pavilion Press.

Turkington, D., Dudley, R., Warman, D.M. and Beck, A.T. (2004) 'Cognitive behaviour therapy for schizophrenia: a review', *Journal of Psychiatric Practice*, 10 (1): 5–16.

Vanstraelen, M., Holt, G. and Bouras, N. (2003) 'Adults with learning disabilities and psychiatric problems', in W. Frazer and M. Kerr (eds), *Seminars in the Psychiatry of Learning Disabilities* (2nd edn). London: Royal College of Psychiatrists.

11

PEOPLE WITH LEARNING DISABILITIES IN THE CRIMINAL JUSTICE SYSTEM

Sarah Campbell and Wendy Goodman

INTRODUCTION

Some people with learning disabilities commit offences and are, therefore, at risk of coming into contact with the criminal justice system; for some this is appropriate but not for all (DH, 2011). Those with mild and borderline learning disabilities account for the majority of the population who have learning disabilities and are less likely to be diverted away from the Criminal Justice System (CJS) than those with more severe learning disabilities (Talbot, 2008). Approximately 1.2 million people in England have a mild to moderate learning disability (DoH, 2001). Extrapolations from prison population figures indicate that every day approximately 5,000 people with learning disabilities are in prison alongside a further 19,500 people with possible borderline learning disabilities (DoH, 2008). A number of documents (see Loucks, 2007; Talbot, 2008; Beebee, 2009; Bradley Report, 2009) have been produced which highlight service deficits, make recommendations, and set standards for the assessment and care of people with learning disabilities within the criminal justice system.

This chapter highlights and discusses the main points for practitioners in health, social services, the criminal justice system and other related agencies to consider when working with people with learning disabilities who offend. It provides practical advice and describes examples of good practice.

A large number of agencies work together to deliver what is known as criminal justice, including the police, the Crown Prosecution Service (CPS), the courts and the National Offender Management Service, which covers the prison and probation services. The purpose of the Criminal Justice System is to deliver justice by detecting crime, convicting and punishing the guilty and helping them to stop future offending. It is also responsible for carrying out the orders of the courts, such as supervising community and custodial orders (www.cjsonline.gov.uk). Twenty to thirty per cent of offenders are thought to have a learning disability or difficulty that is sufficient to hamper their ability to cope with the demands and complexities of the criminal justice system (Loucks, 2007). Hayes et al. (2007) found approximately 7 per cent of inmates in a major UK prison had an IQ below 70, with a further 24 per cent having an IQ between 70 and 79. McBrien et al. (2003) found that 26 per cent of those known to learning disabilities services in one local authority were reported to have offending or risky behaviour and almost 10 per cent had had contact with the criminal justice system at some point in their lives. Therefore, although precise numbers are hard to establish, it is clear that a significant number of offenders have learning disabilities and learning difficulties and until recently their needs had not been fully recognised within either the criminal justice system or within health and social services (Loucks, 2007; Bradley Report, 2009).

People with learning disabilities can be particularly disadvantaged and vulnerable in the criminal justice system. Early identification, provision of appropriate safeguards, use of appropriate communication skills, and effective liaison between agencies are vitally important to ensure that offenders who have learning disabilities are able to proceed through the CJS and be re-established into the community after serving a sentence without undue disadvantage (DH, 2011).

FIRST CONTACT: THE POLICE AND POLICE STATIONS

The police are the first point of contact within the criminal justice system for people who have been accused of a criminal action. When people with a learning disability are arrested the police are required to employ additional safeguards to ensure fair and appropriate treatment. However, police officers may have little training regarding people with learning disabilities and lack understanding of their particular needs. Identifying that a person has a learning disability can be a difficult task and if this is missed, the person is at risk of going through the CJS without having their needs addressed. Some people who are arrested will be known to learning disabilities services and may have paid carers, social workers or health professionals involved in their lives, who alongside family members can help support the individual through the police processes. However, some people arrested by the police may have undiagnosed or unrecognised learning disabilities and may not have access to this support. Or they may have borderline learning disabilities and not be eligible for health and social services support. Police arrest is likely to be a daunting, intimidating and confusing process and people with a learning disability may be particularly vulnerable in this situation. The study by Leggett et al. (2007), examining people with learning disabilities' experiences of being interviewed by the police, illustrates some of the issues from the individual's perspective. One person described how difficult he found it to answer the questions put to him in the police interview: 'Sometimes I couldn't answer the question because I was getting upset and frightened' (direct quotes from service user in Leggett et al., 2007: 172). Another respondent found the police were aware of his difficulties and took care to ensure he was safe in this environment: 'they didn't even lock me in the cell, the door was open and they sat in the cell with me. That was good because I didn't understand why I was there' (direct quotes from service user in Leggett et al., 2007: 172). In this study participants wanted to be listened to, helped to tell their side of the story, and wanted someone who understood their needs.

In order to help protect 'mentally vulnerable' detainees the police follow certain safeguards and procedures as set out in the Police and Criminal Evidence Act of 1984/2006. This Act, with its accompanying Code of Practice, set out the safeguards for 'mentally vulnerable' suspects, which include any detainee who, because of their mental state or capacity, may not understand the significance of the questions they are asked, their replies or other information they give during police processes. The custody officer should err on the side of caution and contact an Appropriate Adult where they have any doubt regarding a detainee's vulnerability. Evidence gained through confession is not admissible in court if the appropriate safeguards were not in place during the police interview.

The main role of the Appropriate Adult is to help prevent unsafe prosecutions. Without the safeguard of an Appropriate Adult, people with a learning disability may be at risk of giving unreliable, misleading or self-incriminating evidence at interview. Prior to interview the Appropriate Adult must explain to the detainee their role, inspect custody records, check that the detainee knows the reason for detention and is aware of their rights (including the right to free legal advice), and make sure the individual understands the procedures. In practice this can be difficult to achieve as many police authorities do not have access to dedicated Appropriate Adult schemes with experience of working with people with learning disabilities. In the absence of Appropriate Adult schemes, social workers and learning disability nurses who know the person may be asked to act in this role. Where the person is unknown to services and learning disability is not confirmed, learning disability services are unlikely to provide an Appropriate Adult. This means the police have limited options when seeking Appropriate Adult provision. An investigation into police responses to suspects with learning disabilities found a number of problems, including inconsistent responses, patchy provision of Appropriate Adults, police difficulties identifying people with learning disabilities, and limited onward referral of suspects to learning disabilities services for further assessment (Jacobson, 2008). The National Appropriate Adult Network (www.appropriateadult.org.uk) provides further information and agreed standards regarding Appropriate Adults.

Reflection Point 31

Do you know who can be an appropriate adult? Do they need any training? If you do not know, ask your colleagues or visit http://www.appropriateadult.org.uk/.

COURTS AND SENTENCING

The criminal courts can be an intimidating arena for any defendant to enter. The language and procedures used are often complex and can be hard to understand and follow. Defendants with a learning disability may benefit from a familiarisation visit to the court before the trial starts. Most people with mild learning disabilities, with appropriate support, will be fit to attend court and enter a plea. If there is doubt about the defendant's fitness to plead the court requires two psychiatric reports to provide an opinion on this. Where a person is not fit to plead, a trial of the facts will take place. The jury then decides whether the defendant committed the act, which is not the same as being found guilty. The court seeks professional advice regarding taking appropriate action if they decide the defendant did commit the act. They may consider using a Guardianship Order (Mental Health Act of 1983/2007), or a section of the Criminal Procedure (Insanity and Unfitness to Plead) Act 1991 if the person requires a period of secure hospital treatment. Civil sections of the Mental Health Act (1983/2007) may also be used. Where the defendant is fit to plead the court proceeds in the usual way but may also seek advice from health and social services on appropriate action to be taken if the person is found guilty.

Scenario

A 40 year old man who was not known to the learning disabilities service was charged with the indecent assault of his 12-year-old niece. The custody sergeant suspected the man had learning disabilities and arranged for an Appropriate Adult to be present during police procedures. The solicitor doubted the man's understanding of the court processes and commissioned a psychological assessment of his intellectual abilities. The psychology report suggested a full scale IQ of 56 and doubted his fitness to plead. The court went on to request two psychiatric assessments which agreed that he was not fit to plead. A trial of the facts occurred and the man was deemed to have committed the acts. He was placed on Guardianship Order with condition that he attend treatment as directed by the Community Learning Disabilities Team psychiatrist and reside as directed by social services. He was provided with a substantial care package, and attended a sex offender treatment group designed for people with learning disabilities.

Points for Good Practice

- Wherever possible people with a mild learning disability should be enabled to go through criminal justice procedures. Appropriate support must be provided
- Expert or professional witnesses at court should liaise with local learning disability professionals in order to ensure that recommendations they make are feasible, realistic and likely to be carried out. For example, if sex offender treatment is recommended efforts should be made to establish its local availability.

COURT LIAISON

Court liaison services have developed across the UK and in Australia and while there has been limited research into their effectiveness, reports have indicated improvements in links between criminal justice and health and social services resulting in improved outcomes for vulnerable people (Sharples et al., 2003; Kingham and Corfe, 2005). The Cross Government Strategy – Mental Health Division Report, *New Horizons: A Shared Vision for Mental Health* (2009) discusses the Court Liaison Services and highlights that the NHS contract from 2010 will include meeting the needs of people with learning disabilities in the Criminal Justice System.

Court liaison services are based in the courts and provide screening, initial assessments, advice to the courts and liaison with local services where a defendant is suspected of having significant mental health problems. They aim to provide the court with useful and timely information regarding the defendant's mental state, advise on communication approaches and potential care pathway, and where possible diverting people who have mental illness from custodial sentences into appropriate community settings where therapeutic interventions can be provided.

The court assessment and referral service based in Bristol Magistrates' Court has access to a learning disability nurse who works alongside the mental health team. The role involves initial assessments of those appearing in court who are identified as possibly having learning disabilities, providing the court with timely advice, liaison with local learning disability services, follow-up assessment, and following up those who are remanded or sentenced to prison. However, while good practice, the involvement of learning disabilities nurses in court liaison services appears patchy. Therefore, good liaison between local learning disability services, court and prison healthcare staff is key to gathering information regarding the individuals' needs, the appropriate care pathway and whether specific assessments would be helpful. In the absence of this information and input from the local learning disability service it seems more likely that inappropriate actions might be taken, including lengthy remand to prison awaiting specialist assessments that might not always be necessary.

PROBATION AND COMMUNITY ORDERS

The national probation service provides pre-sentence reports to advise the courts on sentencing convicted offenders. It also supervises offenders in the community on specific court orders and those released on license from prison. The probation service aims to protect the public, reduce re-offending, rehabilitate offenders, and enhance their awareness of the effects of crime on victims and communities (National Probation Service, 2002). Although there are some adapted probation programmes, not all programmes have been adapted to meet the needs of people with learning disabilities (DH, 2011). Where programmes do not meet needs there is scope for probation and learning disability services to work jointly on the treatment of offenders who have learning disabilities (DH, 2011). Probation programmes are expected to maintain programme integrity, with group facilitators carefully following the manual (see National Probation Service, 2002). A more flexible approach is generally needed when working with offenders who have learning disabilities, for example material may need to be presented in a number of different ways and repeated often in order for the participant to understand and recall information. A number of detailed treatment manuals have been developed for people with learning disabilities, which may be suitable for use with people who have come into conflict with the criminal justice system. Some programmes address issues related to anger and violence, while others concentrate on sexual offending (Sinclair et al., 2002; Taylor and Novaco, 2005; Blasingame, 2006; O'Neil, 2006). Examples of successful therapeutic community programmes include The Good Thinking Programme and The Men's Group:

The 'Good Thinking' Programme   This was developed by the Avon Forensic Community Learning Disabilities Team to meet the needs of people with learning disabilities. The programme is based on the premise that offending behaviour is an anti-social means of attaining an appropriate goal. The course aims to enable participants to develop pro-social means to attain their goals. It includes helping participants to identify achievable goals, developing social skills including assertiveness and perspective taking skills, emotion recognition and a basic problem solving strategy. Many participants attend as a condition of a probation order and this requires close collaboration between services. The course comprises 25 sessions of two hours on a weekly basis and lasts six months. Generally, the feedback has been positive from those who finish the course and a variety of learning disabilities services nationally, including inpatient services, are running or plan to run this course.

The Men's Group   This nationally evaluated programme (Murphy and Sinclair, 2007) was developed by the Sex Offender Treatment Services Collaborative – Intellectual Disability to provide treatment for men with learning disabilities who are at risk of sexual offending (University of Kent, 2010). Several clinical teams run this programme nationally, with each team adapting their material to the needs of the service user group. The Men's Group meets for two hours on a weekly basis and lasts between twelve and eighteen months. It comprises five modules, including sex education, the cognitive-behavioural model, the four-stage model of sexual offending, victim empathy and relapse prevention. The expectation is that participants develop their own individualised relapse prevention or staying safe plan before the course has ended. Courses are evaluated through the use of psychological measures, feedback from the participants and their support services, and changes in behaviour or re-offending rates.

Therapeutic groups aim to enable offenders who have learning disabilities to develop their sense of responsibility for their actions and learn strategies to keep themselves from future offending. However, it would be unrealistic to expect that attending a treatment programme alone would be sufficient to significantly reduce the risk of re-offending. Where people's lives are impoverished and lack good housing, employment, positive relationships and opportunities for meaningful daily activity it is extremely unlikely that individuals will be able to make significant changes to their lives and reduce their risk of offending without substantial support from services. Therapeutic work is just one component of a multi-agency approach that includes working jointly with probation services. This ensures offending behaviours are taken seriously and enable people who have learning disability to take responsibility for their actions, while at the same time receiving appropriate support. Joint working also:

- Encourages clear, open communication regarding roles, expectations and sharing of information
- Prevents or reduces risk of imprisonment, helping individuals to stay in the community
- Opens up opportunities to benefit from other services offered by Community Learning Disabilities Teams including Health Action Plans and skills assessments.

PRISON AND PRISON HEALTHCARE

Being given a custodial sentence is stressful and can be a frightening and confusing experience. Much of the information available in the form of leaflets and posters is in a written format that requires the person reading it to have a reasonable reading age (usually 8–10 years). In 2009 the Department of Health and the Prison Reform Trust issued two booklets aimed at prisoners with disabilities. The books give people with a disability coming into prison an insight into prison life and details about where to go for help. Copies of the booklets are available through the Prison Reform Trust, prison library, Disability Liaison Officers (a statutory requirement in all prisons) and the prison healthcare team. There is also the prison service website which has a section that enables the internet user to take a virtual tour of prison life, including the reception process. This is valuable as a visual resource for people to see what the inside of a prison is like and the processes to expect.

The Grubin Health Screen is a statutory document that must be completed for every person on reception into prison (Grubin et al., 1999; Grubin et al., 2002; Ministry of Justice National Offender Management Service, 2010). The screening includes data on blood pressure, pulse, temperature and general health history. This is followed by a secondary health screen (within 48 hours of their arrival) to offer any immunisations, sexual health, blood borne virus screening and chronic disease investigations which may be appropriate as a result of the initial health screen. Those people known to have a learning disability are referred to the in-reach team and remain on their caseloads while in prison. In-reach teams liaise with the relevant community learning disability team for background information and continuity of care. There is a care pathway to ensure that they are not 'lost' while in custody. The Department of Health is examining the current role of the in-reach teams to ensure they are providing services for those with severe mental illness. This should involve the development of liaison and diversion services to undertake some of the current non-clinical activities (Bradley Report, 2009).

One of the main issues for staff working in prison is recognising when a person has learning disabilities. Prison staff may have limited knowledge and experience of people with learning disabilities and may lack understanding regarding the communication and support needs of this group. Prison teams and local learning disability services need to establish and maintain links to promote recognition and understanding of people who have learning disabilities. Examples of good practice involving learning disabilities nurses working in prison healthcare teams exist, however, such good practice is often reliant upon individual practitioners' interest and commitment (Beebee, 2009).

Reflection Point 32

Developing good practice often involves people who have good networking skills and who build relationships across organisations. Whom do you know who supports offenders who have learning disabilities? Map out these people. Your map should include (if they exist) court liaison staff with a learning disability remit, local forensic learning disability teams, Community Learning Disabilities Team (CLDT) contacts, drug and alcohol services, local prison nursing staff, any learning disability nurses employed in the prison, and your local probation team contacts.

The prison day is repetitive and sticks rigidly to a timetable that may be helpful to some people with learning disabilities. However, in order for people to be able to make sense of what is happening around them, more needs to be done to promote alternative communication, such as pictorial signs and symbols to help people understand their environment, for example pictorial daily menus.

People with learning disabilities are also vulnerable to exploitation and bullying (DH, 2011) and staff need to be vigilant when observing prisoners carrying out their activities of daily living. People with a learning disability may need support with collecting their meals, keeping their cells and themselves clean, and accessing their phone calls, visits and mail. Prison in-reach teams are the main vehicle for improvements in mental health services for prisoners, especially those with severe and enduring mental illness. Established ten years ago across all prisons they ensure that the needs of those with severe and enduring mental illness are met and that the transfer to an appropriate secondary care health facility is achieved as soon as possible, if this is appropriate (Steel et al., 2007). Although mental health nurses work in prison healthcare and it is best practice for the mental health teams to work across the primary and complex mental health spectrum, there appears to be no research on how these teams are including people with learning disabilities in the criminal justice system.

Scenario

Mr B was remanded to a local prison where he was located on the Vulnerable Persons wing being subject to Rule 45 because of his alleged offences. (Rule 45 is offered to those prisoners whose alleged offences may put them at risk from other prisoners; they are located separately from other prisoners and hence are protected from any assault.) Mr B remained in the local prison for eight months without giving staff any reason to be concerned about his level of functioning or coping skills. After a routine court appearance, Mr B was received at the local prison and was assessed in reception by a mental health nurse who completed a brief assessment looking at Mr B's physical and mental health. The nurse also completed the brief questionnaire aimed at getting the assessor to consider the prisoner's ability to engage with the reception process.

The way Mr B answered the questions highlighted that Mr B may have a learning disability. At this point the reception nurse referred Mr B to the prison in-reach team who made enquiries about any services which Mr B may have received in the past. The healthcare team, in-reach team and court diversion service worked together to complete reports for the Judge overseeing Mr B's case. Mr B was seen by two psychiatrists during his stay and a care package arranged whereby Mr B was transferred under Section 38 of the Mental Health Act 1983 to a local specialist assessment and rehabilitation service for people with a learning disability.

During his stay at the local specialist unit Mr B received a full and comprehensive assessment of his level of functioning and his needs. He also had regular sessions with a specialist psychologist who was able to work with Mr B on his offending behaviour, helping to reduce his ongoing level of risk. This was viewed very positively by the Judge and at his next court hearing Mr B was sentenced to a probation order with a comprehensive care package in the community.

POSITIVE OUTCOMES

The use by the reception nurse of the questionnaire identifying Mr B's possible learning disabilities is one of a number of strategies that enabled this positive outcome to occur. The Learning Disabilities Screening Questionnaire has been found to be a useful tool and is being used in many prisons to improve identification of people who have a learning disability (DH, 2011). In the scenario above it prompted referral to the prison in-reach team and ultimately court diversion to an environment where Mr B could receive risk and functional assessments that enabled him to recognise what his triggers were and how to avoid situations involving those risks in the future. The process also ensured that Mr B received ongoing monitoring and support in the community. The whole process involved various services communicating and working together to create a pathway for Mr B, which encompassed his health needs but also addressed his offending behaviour, thus reducing his ongoing risk levels to the general public. Staff at the specialist assessment and habilitation unit were initially daunted by the prospect of having a man of Mr B's intellectual ability and offending history in their care. The team did not feel that they had the skills to provide the assessment and manage the risks that Mr B might pose in the community. A mental health nurse from the prison attended a staff meeting at the unit to discuss these issues with the staff team. This proved invaluable for the unit staff and went some way to allay any anxieties they were experiencing regarding Mr B's care.

The Bradley Report (2009) states that all judiciary staff should receive learning disability awareness training and this should extend to prison staff. The *Prison Health Performance and Quality Indicators* (DH, 2009) are reviewed every six months and assessed yearly and they include a specific quality indicator relating to the care of people with learning disabilities in custody. This includes learning disability awareness training for staff to involve local Community Learning Disability Teams and service users in delivery of the training.

Reflection Point 33

How can you be involved in improving staff knowledge of people with learning disabilities? Depending on your own role, could you do one of the following activities to promote an increase in your and others knowledge?

Offering to provide awareness training to local prison staff

Requesting awareness training from your manager

Commissioning training from a local CLDT

Giving a short talk about what you have learnt from your reading.

LEAVING PRISON

When people with a learning disability are received into prison an annual health check and Health Action Plan (HAP) should follow them into custody. Where there is no HAP, a health check is carried out and a HAP created and shared with criminal justice and health agencies upon discharge, as necessary. Projects such as those run by the Prince's Trust (2011) and Supporting Others through Volunteer Action (SOVA) (2010) are increasing access to mentorship for those leaving prison. The mentor might help to arrange housing, benefits and employment or provide support groups as appropriate. Help to access healthcare, such as registering with a doctor, should be arranged with pre-release engagement workers working with mentors to ensure the individual's needs are met. Pre-release engagement workers have local knowledge of, and connections with, statutory and non-statutory organisations and work to ensure that people can be signposted to appropriate services on release from prison. The role includes working with the prisoner prior to release, liaison with services and follow up after release.

General Advice for Criminal Justice Personnel

- Find out about your local Community Learning Disabilities Team
- Make contact, invite them to your team meeting or invite yourself to theirs
- Develop your knowledge of learning disability; perhaps identify people in the team who can develop specialist knowledge in this area
- Be flexible with your communication skills in order to find the best way to make yourself understood
- Always thoroughly check that the person has understood what you have said and the information given to them
- Ask the individual the best way to give them information and then do it that way
- Pursue joint working with others involved.

General Advice for Learning Disability Services

- Find out about your local probation team, police station and prison health staff
- Make contact; ask if you can attend a team meeting to introduce your service
- Offer and encourage training on working and communicating with people who have learning disabilities

- Learn what you can about the criminal justice system and how you can help support people with learning disabilities who enter this system
- If a service user goes to prison, don't discharge them. Contact prison healthcare and arrange to visit them. Provide advice regarding care, approaches and communication. Check that health needs are being met and ensure a care pathway is in place before their release date
- The Prison Health Quality Performance Indicators for 2010–2011 state that all those in prison for longer than twelve months with a learning disability must have a health action plan in place.

CONCLUSION

There is a developing body of work, including research and government guidance, which aims to address the needs of people with learning disabilities who come into contact with the criminal justice system. The Prison Reform Trust through *No-One Knows* (Talbot, 2008) enabled service users to share their experiences of different aspects of the system including arrest, going to court and prison. The main themes arising from the work include lack of structured identification of learning disability, lack of accessible information, need to increase multi-agency working and planning, need to address disability discrimination, and workforce development issues, including raising awareness of learning disability and inclusion of learning disabilities staff within prison healthcare settings. The *No-One Knows* project influenced the findings and recommendations of the Bradley Report (2009) in relation to the needs of offenders with learning disabilities. In community and secure hospital settings clinical staff have developed offender treatment programmes specifically for people with learning disabilities, some of whom work closely with probation services to ensure that, where possible and appropriate, people with a learning disability remain in the community and access therapeutic services rather than serve custodial sentences. Further work is needed to ensure that prisoners with learning disabilities have equitable access to treatment programmes in prison.

The Bradley Report advocates early identification and assessment of people with mental health problems and learning disabilities when they come into contact with the criminal justice system. The prison estate across the UK aims to introduce a simple screening tool for learning disability on reception to prison, however, with greater learning disability practitioner presence in police and court settings it is envisaged that those going through the criminal justice system will be highlighted as having a possible learning disability earlier on in the system. There is a developing role in police stations, courts, prisons and community settings for learning disabilities practitioners to use their specialist skills with this vulnerable group of people. In addition, there is a significant number of people in the criminal justice system who have learning difficulties and struggle with the complexity of the system. These people will not necessarily meet the criteria for learning disabilities services but have similar needs in terms of communication, understanding processes and being vulnerable to others. However, if processes change to accommodate people with learning disabilities this should also be helpful to those with learning difficulties and others with reduced cognitive functioning. The key to good practice when working with offenders who have learning disabilities is good liaison with a wide range of services and the willingness to persevere and adopt a flexible approach in order to meet individual needs.

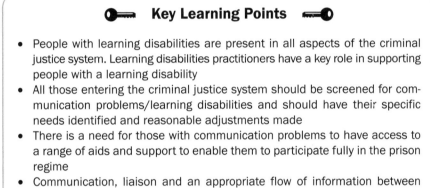

🔑 Key Learning Points 🔑

- People with learning disabilities are present in all aspects of the criminal justice system. Learning disabilities practitioners have a key role in supporting people with a learning disability
- All those entering the criminal justice system should be screened for communication problems/learning disabilities and should have their specific needs identified and reasonable adjustments made
- There is a need for those with communication problems to have access to a range of aids and support to enable them to participate fully in the prison regime
- Communication, liaison and an appropriate flow of information between agencies is key to ensuring a joint approach to meeting the needs of offenders with learning disabilities
- All teams working with offenders with learning disabilities should map out other relevant agencies in their area and make contact.

REFERENCES

Beebee, J. (2009) *A Mapping Exercise into Service Provision for People with Learning Disabilities who have Offended or are at Risk Offending (Interim Report).* Weston-Super-Mare: NHS South West Offender Health.

Blasingame, G.D. (2006) *Working with Forensic Clients with Severe and Sexual Behaviour Problems: Practical Treatment Strategies for Persons with Intellectual Disabilities.* Oklahoma: Wood 'N' Barnes.

Bradley Report (2009) *The Bradley Report: Lord Bradley's Review of People with Mental Health Problems or Learning Disabilities in the Criminal Justice System.* London: Department of Health.

Criminal Procedure (Insanity and Unfitness to Plead) Act (1991) London: HMSO.

Cross Government Strategy – Mental Health Division (2009) *New Horizons: A Shared Vision for Mental Health*. London: Department of Health.

Department of Health (2001) *Valuing People: A New Strategy for Learning Disability for the 21st Century*. London: Department of Health.

Department of Health (2008) *Offender Health and Social Care Strategy Data Report*. London: Department of Health.

Department of Health (2009) *Guidance Notes: Prison Health Performance and Quality Indicators*. London: Department of Health.

Department of Health (2011) *Positive Practice Positive Outcome: A Handbook for Professionals in the Criminal Justice System Working with Offenders with Learning Disabilities*. London: Department Of Health.

Department of Health and Prison Reform Trust (2009) *Information Book for Prisoners with a Disability*. London: Prison Reform Trust.

Grubin, D., Parsons. S. and Hopkins, C. (1999) *Report on the Evaluation of a New Reception Health Questionnaire and Associated Training*. London: Her Majesty's Prison Service.

Grubin, D., Carson, D. and Parsons, S. (2002) *Report on New Reception Health Screening Arrangements: The Result of a Pilot Study in 10 Prisons*. London: Department of Health.

Hayes. S., Shackell, P., Mottram, P. and Lancaster, R. (2007) 'The prevalence of intellectual disabilities in a major UK prison', *British Journal of Learning Disabilities*, 35: 162–7.

Jacobson, J. (2008) *Police Responses to Suspects with Learning Disabilities and Learning Difficulties: A Review of Policy and Practice*. London: Prison Reform Trust.

Kingham, M. and Corfe, M. (2005) 'Experiences of a mixed court liaison and diversion scheme', *Psychiatric Bulletin*, 29: 137–40.

Leggett, J., Goodman, W. and Dinani, S. (2007) 'People with learning disabilities' experiences of being interviewed by the police', *British Journal of Learning Disabilities*, 35 (3): 168–73.

Loucks, N. (2007) *No-One Knows: Offenders with Learning Difficulties and Learning Disabilities – Review of Prevalence and Associated Needs*. London: Prison Reform Trust.

McBrien, J., Hodgetts, A. and Gregory, J. (2003) 'Offending and risky behaviour in community services for people with intellectual disabilities in one local authority', *Journal of Forensic Psychiatry and Psychology*, 14: 280–97.

Mental Health Act (1983/2007) London: HMSO.

Ministry of Justice National Offender Management Service (2010) *PSI 052 Early Days in Custody – Reception, First Night and Induction*. London: Ministry of Justice National Offender Management Service.

Murphy, G.H. and Sinclair, N. (2007) *Effectiveness of Cognitive-Behavioural Treatment for Men with Learning Disabilities at Risk of Sexual Offending: Final Report to the Department of Health*. London: Department of Health.

National Probation Service (2002) *National Management Manual for Effective Delivery of Accredited Programmes in the Community (V2)*. London: Home Office.

O'Neil, H. (2006) *Managing Anger*. Chichester: John Wiley and Sons.

Police and Criminal Evidence Act (1984/2006). London: HMSO.

Prince's Trust (2011) *Helping Change Young Lives*. [online] Available from http://www.princes-trust.org.uk/about_the_trust/what_we_do/programmes/leaving_prison_mentoring.aspx, accessed 04.04.2011.

Sharples, J., Lewin, T., Hinton, R., Sly, K., Coles, G., Johnston, P. and Carr, V. (2003) 'Offending behaviour and mental illness: characteristics of a mental health court liaison service', *Psychiatry, Psychology and Law*, 10 (2): 300–15.

Sinclair, N., Booth, S.J. and Murphy, G. (2002) *Cognitive Behavioural Treatment for Men with Intellectual Disabilities who are at Risk of Sexual Offending: A Treatment Manual Prepared for the Sex Offender Treatment South East Collaborative – Intellectual Disability (SOTSEC-ID)*. Kent: Tizard Centre.

Steel, J., Thornicroft, G., Birmingham, L., Brooker, C., Mills, A., Harty, M. and Shaw, J. (2007) 'Prison mental health inreach services', *The British Journal of Psychiatry*, 190: 373–4.

Supporting Others through Volunteer Action (SOVA) (2010) *Annual Review 2009–2010*. London: Supporting Others through Volunteer Action.

Talbot, J. (2008) *Prisoners' Voices: Experiences of the Criminal Justice System by Prisoners with Learning Disabilities and Difficulties*. London: Prison Reform Trust.

Taylor, J.L. and Novaco, R. (2005) *Anger Treatment for People with Developmental Disabilities: A Theory, Evidence and Manual Based Approach*. Chichester: John Wiley and Sons.

University of Kent (2010) *Sex Offender Treatment Services Collaborative – Intellectual Disability*. [online] Available from http://www.kent.ac.uk/tizard/sotsec/index.html, accessed 25.03.2011.

12 PROFESSIONAL PRACTICE

Crispin Hebron

INTRODUCTION

This chapter explores professional practice and its importance in relation to meeting the health and social care needs of people with learning disabilities. The concept of professionalism is explored and then set in the current policy context impacting on professional practice with people with learning disabilities. Codes of conduct are discussed, compared and the common themes identified. Professional practice with people with learning disabilities is then considered against this backdrop in terms of judgements, decision making, consent and ethical practice and confidentiality.

PROFESSIONALISM

Professionalism is not easily defined. Morrell (2003) summarised Downie's (1990) proposed six characteristics of professionals as follows:

1   Professionals have skills or expertise proceeding from a broad knowledge base
2   Professionals provide a service based on a special relationship with those whom he or she serves. This relationship involves a special attitude of beneficence tempered with integrity. This includes fairness, honesty and a bond based on legal and ethical rights and duties authorised by the professional institution and legalised by public esteem
3   To the extent that the public recognises the authority of the professional, he or she has the social function of speaking out on broad matters of public policy and justice, going beyond duties to specific clients

4   In order to discharge these functions, professionals must be independent of the influence of the State or commerce
5   The professional should be educated rather than trained. This means having a wide cognitive perspective, seeing the place of his or her skills within that perspective and continuing to develop this knowledge and skills within a framework of values
6   A professional should have legitimised authority. If a profession is to have credibility in the eyes of the general public, it must be widely recognised as independent, disciplined by its professional association, actively expanding its knowledge base and concerned with the education of its members. If it is widely recognised as satisfying these conditions, then it will possess moral as well as legal legitimacy, and its pronouncements will be listened to with respect.' (Morrell, 2003)

It is interesting to compare this list with the common themes identified from various codes of conduct discussed later in the chapter. Autonomy is central to professionalism, in that a profession is given the right to control its own work by determining who can do the work and how the work should be done. From this flows self-regulation, the authority delegated by the state to a profession to determine standards of conduct, practice and training, and to regulate entry to the profession and continuing practice.

While it is important to have an understanding of professionalism within a profession, practitioners also need to be able to interpret that understanding into everyday action. Professionals need to understand what professionalism means in their everyday work. A useful framework to remember and apply is to think of professionalism in practice as the bringing together of professional behaviours, attitudes and beliefs. It is important not to be obsessed with our outward behaviours at the expense of our attitudes and beliefs. The three must be understood and considered in relation to each other; beliefs are the causes of our attitudes, which in turn cause our behaviours.

THE POLICY CONTEXT OF PROFESSIONAL PRACTICE

Modern professional practice is set in a rapidly developing policy context. Not only is it important for practitioners to be professionally responsive to policy direction but additionally to utilise such awareness as a framework in which to respond effectively to the needs of some of the most vulnerable people in society. The development of policy that either includes people with learning disabilities or specifically addresses the inequalities present within the population has burgeoned over the past decade. It is interesting to note that many of the underpinning drivers of current mainstream policy development are already established and familiar in professional learning disability practice; personalisation, choice, equalities, inclusion, health action planning, and person centredness are all good examples now seen in cross cutting health and social care policy. This amounts to a commitment to care for all, including people with learning disabilities, based on individual need – shaping services around needs of individual patients, families and carers and reducing inequalities.

This policy context places an onus on organisations, teams and, ultimately, individual practitioners to embrace these elements of service delivery and develop enabling practices. Professional practitioners will increasingly find themselves supporting people with learning disabilities in a range of settings and will need continually to challenge and develop their own practice to meet this demand. This is due to not only the inclusive nature of current policy but also to other factors:

- people with learning disabilities are living longer, leading to more age-related diseases such as stroke, heart disease, respiratory disease and cancer
- there is an increasing number of young people with severe and profound disabilities and associated complex health needs.

Additionally, people with learning disabilities are more likely to:

- experience mental illness
- experience chronic health problems including epilepsy
- have physical and sensory impairment
- experience poverty
- be socially isolated
- have poor oral health which can lead to chronic dental disease. (Bernal, 2005)

The focus on health acknowledges its status as a key factor in improving quality of life and social inclusion. Improving health and access to health-care remains central to improving the lives of people with learning disabilities, the overall objective being to enable people with learning disabilities to access a health service designed around their individual needs, with fast and convenient care delivered to a consistently high standard and with additional support where necessary.

Disability Equality Duty and Reasonable Adjustments

Since December 2006 there has been a legal duty on public sector organisations to promote equality of opportunity and outcome for people with disabilities. Public service providers need to evidence, as part of their disability equality duty, that they provide services to all people irrespective of their disability and, as part of their risk management standards, clarify how they care for people who are deemed vulnerable. This requires services and practitioners to make reasonable adjustments to ensure that each person has the same opportunity and equality of outcome, whether they have a learning disability or not (Disability Discrimination Act 1995, amended 2006). This could mean for example GPs and practice staff offering longer appointments, providing accessible information and taking carers' concerns seriously (Michael Report, 2008). There is a need for practitioners to consider how they respond individually to the needs of each person with a learning disability to deliver person centred care. Disability discrimination legislation has further been strengthened by the Equality Act, which became law in the autumn of 2010.

Inclusion and Professional Practice

The Office of Disability Issues (2010) identifies that the disabilities and experiences of individuals are often much more to do with society's attitudes, the environment and the way organisations operate than any original impairment. If services and individual practitioners are to have a positive impact on the quality of life of people with learning disabilities then an understanding of this social model of disability, citizenship and social inclusion are vital. A traditional medical approach to the needs of people with learning disabilities is no longer adequate; the use of the medical model has pathologised and objectified people with intellectual disabilities leading to them being seen as 'less human' (Klotz, 2004). Services and service systems pose dangers when both professionals and society fail to demonstrate positive values and ethics to ensure the protection of people with learning disabilities within systems of care, as clearly demonstrated by Mencap in their *Death by Indifference* report (2007). Both systems and practice reforms need to be guided by understanding of social approaches to disability; not only from professionals but from society itself. Such wisdom and understanding is generated from the inherited values and social ethics of a society, and reflected in professional activity. A modern professional approach to practice has the power to influence and promote greater understanding of the marginalisation of vulnerable people, including those with learning disabilities, and bring about improvements through the ongoing development of social modelling (Hunter and Kendrick, 2009). Modern professional practice therefore brings the need to understand and relate to the complexity of human health and well-being and consider how social, psychological and biological factors interact in the construction of health and quality of life (Duggan et al., 2002).

The policy emphasis is now firmly on more social issues of rights and responsibilities, social inclusion and citizenship: but there are potential hazards. Moves away from a biomedical model of disability towards a social model must not deflect attention and resources away from the known health inequalities (Emerson and Baines, 2010) of the learning disability population. This is particularly important as the proportion of people with profound and multiple disabilities living into adulthood has increased in the last twenty years, as has the number of those with complex challenges such as autism (Emerson, 2009; Mansell, 2010). Professional practice focusses on bringing about positive outcomes for individuals and groups. Quality of life is, arguably, the most important outcome measure for people with learning disabilities. Quality of life is made up of many aspects, including physical, material, and emotional health and well-being, as well as interpersonal relationships, personal development, self-determination, social inclusion, and civic rights. People with learning disabilities are likely to experience poorer outcomes in all of these areas. The RCN's professional development guidance (Royal College of Nursing, 2011) on learning disabilities highlights the link between social exclusion and such inequalities.

Within the learning disabled population itself there are groups who face even greater barriers and potential discrimination. For example, those who show challenging behaviour often make other people uncomfortable so that social inclusion is more difficult, and evidence suggests that both children and adults with learning disabilities and challenging behaviour (and their families) have a poorer quality of life and more restrictions in their lives than others with learning disabilities (Murphy, 2009). Similarly, people with profound and multiple learning disabilities (PMLD) are frequently excluded through a lack of understanding of their individual needs. It is only through professionalism, determined efforts and dedication from practitioners that such barriers can be reduced. A recent volume by Pawlyn and Carnaby (2009) dedicated to the nursing needs of people with PMLD expertly describes the strength of professional feeling and expertise behind this philosophical and ethical stand.

Reflection Point 34

Reflect on a recent experience you may have of receiving a service; identify the aspects that worked well for you and those that needed to be improved.

Now think about somebody with a learning disability and consider how they might have experienced the same service.

List what would need to be done differently (reasonable adjustments) for the policy direction of inclusion described above to be made a reality for people with a learning disability.

Professional Practice with People with Learning Disabilities – Codes of Conduct

Codes of Conduct regulate and govern individual professional practices that are implemented through professional membership of professional councils. The environment in which all codes of conduct operate is complex, involving difficult decisions and complicated choices. The term 'Duty of Care' is often used as a rule of thumb, which means making the care of people the prime concern, treating them as individuals and respecting their dignity. The Nursing and Midwifery Council (NMC) Code of Conduct (2008: 1) identifies trust and the justification of that trust as central to professional practice. The General Social Care Council (GSCC) (2010) and the Health Professions Council (HPC) (2008) – who currently regulate fourteen health professions including art therapists, chiropodists, dieticians, occupational therapists, paramedics, physiotherapists, radiographers and speech and language therapists – offer similar frameworks to guide professional practice. This regulatory and governance approach, familiar in professional domains, is now increasingly apparent in the management of delivering services through professional practice with a *Code of Conduct for NHS Managers* now established (DoH, 2002). While professional and management practices are often perceived as being derived from differing bases the similarities are marked, with striking commonalities between the codes of conduct. Table 12.1 compares examples from healthcare, social care and management to draw out these commonalities.

These common themes are central to successfully and safely meeting the needs of any individual and while not taken for granted are often tacitly or subconsciously applied. However, for people with learning disabilities they represent aspects of their lives that have often been overlooked or ignored because of the complexity of their needs or through negative assumptions from practitioners and society. They are the fundamental principles on which to base any approach to a person with a learning disability and provide a solid framework for professional practice.

Trust and Integrity

For people with learning disabilities trust needs to be established on an individual basis, requiring an understanding of each individual. Issues such as communication, capacity, previous experiences, history and existing levels of support need consideration.

TABLE 12.1 Codes of Conduct – Comparisons and Commonalities from Healthcare, Social Care and Management Codes

Common themes	Trust and integrity	Rights, dignity and respect	Evidence based practice and standards	Learning	Autonomy and accountability	Safety
Health care NMC (2008) HPC (2008)	Working with others to protect and promote the health and well-being of individuals, families, carers, and the wider community	Providing a high standard of practice and care at all times	Being open and honest, acting with integrity and upholding the reputation of the profession	Keep your professional knowledge up to date	Respecting confidentiality	Acting within the limits of your knowledge, skills and experience and, if necessary, refer the matter to another practitioner
Social care GSCC (2010)	Strive to establish and maintain the trust and confidence of service users and carers	Uphold public trust and confidence in social care services	Respect the rights of service users while seeking to ensure that their behaviour does not harm them or other people	Promote the independence of service users while protecting them as far as possible from danger or harm	Be accountable for the quality of their work and take responsibility for maintaining and improving their knowledge and skills	Protect the rights and promote the interests of service users and carers
Managerial NHS Managers (DoH, 2002)	Being honest and acting with integrity	Respecting the public, patients, relatives, carers, NHS staff and partners in other agencies	Showing commitment to working as a team member by working with all colleagues in the NHS and the wider community	Taking responsibility for your own learning and development	Accepting responsibility for your own work and the proper performance of the people you manage	Making the care and safety of patients the first concern and acting to protect them from risk

Dignity and Respect

Dignity is a multi-faceted concept and can be interpreted in different ways. The RCN offers the following definition:

> Dignity is concerned with how people feel, think and behave in relation to the worth or value of themselves and others. To treat someone with dignity is to treat them as a being of worth, in a way that is respectful of them as valued individuals. (2008: 8)

Dignity for people with learning disabilities often involves what other people may take for granted, for example asking the person what they want, what support they need and including the individual at all stages of the care planning process. This may involve taking more time to prepare and using alternative or additional communication methods (see below and Chapter 7).

Evidence Based Practice

All professional codes of practice require practitioners to maintain up–to-date standards of practice and provide evidence based care. For work with individuals with learning disabilities, this requires a synergy of evidence from mainstream practice and from the learning disability field, set alongside individual experience and skills. This requires a dynamic approach to practice that will lead to truly individualised care and support with meaningful outcomes.

Learning

It is essential that professional practice is carried out within a culture of learning and development, both on an individual and organisational level. Any work with people with learning disabilities will present learning opportunities that can influence practice and help improve individuals' experiences of care. The transferring of learning through reflective approaches offers opportunities to develop professional practice and improve the health and well-being of both individuals and the wider learning disabled population.

Autonomy

Aspects of autonomy include self-determination, independence, self-regulation and self-realisation. Autonomy requires dual consideration as it is an important professional aspect in decision making and has become an increasingly important issue for people with learning disabilities. However, despite the policy emphasis on promoting autonomy, the exercise of autonomy in relation to health has so far rarely been an issue in the literature (Wullink et al., 2009).

Accountability

Accountability is integral to professional practice; any registered practitioner is accountable for their professional actions at all times. Accountability is being answerable for one's own judgements and actions, not only to an appropriate person or authority but importantly to individuals in receipt of professional care. This again is an area of particular importance because practitioners are no less accountable to someone with a learning disability than to any citizen. It is worth reflecting on this as the many examples of professionals failing people with learning disabilities can be traced back to this point (Parliamentary and Health Service Ombudsman, 2009). Practitioners make judgements in a wide variety of circumstances, using their professional knowledge, judgement and skills to make a decision based on evidence for best practice and the person's best interests; along with this goes the requirement to justify all the decisions made. The NMC Code says, 'As a professional, you are personally accountable for actions and omissions in your practice and must always be able to justify your decisions' (NMC, 2008: 1).

Safety

The issue of safety is particularly poignant for people with learning disabilities as the risks associated with professional practices are often magnified by the complexity of individuals' needs and exacerbated by communication difficulties. Codes of conduct also offer specific guidance on the delegation of care to others such as care support staff, relatives or other professionals, requiring professionals to take responsibility for delegating any aspect of care.

Networks

Collaborative and partnership working are essential to ensuring evidence based practice and support is available. This establishes the role of networks and professional communication as crucial to successfully meeting the needs of people with learning disabilities in all practice settings. Networking is a dynamic way of establishing and using contacts for information, support and other assistance (Benton, 1997), providing governance regimes and the development of a culture of mutual cooperation (Junki, 2006), along with opportunities for Continued Professional Development. Networks can be based on information sharing, care coordinating or clinical management, and they may be formal or informal. Howarth (2006) provides comprehensive guidance on the activities required to develop, manage and maintain networks. The key benefits to networking are:

- the opportunity to explore issues relating to the scope of professional practice
- reducing social and professional isolation
- a mutually supportive environment in which to develop professional practice
- opportunities for Continued Professional Development.

The development of local and national professional networks provides the vehicle to achieve the objectives of equal access and outcome for people with learning disabilities in mainstream services. This requires all practitioners to strive towards open and transparent working practices where account-ability to individuals with a learning disability is the impetus for continuous improvement.

Reflection Point 35

Write down a list of beliefs or values that you have about your professional practice (these may well be reflected in the codes of conduct already dis-cussed, such as honesty or confidentiality). Now, thinking about how this affects your professional attitudes write a list of the behaviours (the things you do while at work) that demonstrate those beliefs.

PROFESSIONAL APPROACHES WITH PEOPLE WITH LEARNING DISABILITIES

Having explored what constitutes professional practice, in the context of current policy and thinking, and drawn out the key themes from various codes of conduct, this now needs to be applied to professional practice directly with people with learning disabilities. By applying the commonly held principles of the codes of conduct in positive, constructive and some-times innovative ways means practitioners can have a huge impact on an individual's quality of life, through improving access to services, the effec-tiveness of interventions, improving an individual's safety and well-being, and their experience of receiving good care and support.

Accessing Appropriate Services and Assessment

The focus of achieving equitable health and well-being for people with learning disabilities is clearly established as being through mainstream services such as primary and acute health services or local authority provision, with support and specialist input from learning disability services (DH, 2008). This significant shift brings with it certain responsibilities for practitioners in all settings to be confident that they can apply the same professional standards to their practice with individuals with learning disabilities as with the general population. Providing good quality care for people with learning disabilities involves more than just a brief assessment of presenting problems.

Professional assessment needs to be a proactive, structured process that addresses the generic and specific needs of each individual, while allowing appropriate referral to specialist services.

Assessment in a health setting provides a good illustration. As discussed in previous chapters, people with learning disabilities experience a range of conditions, which in the general population would normally be self-presented to their GP but without self-reporting or carer recognition go untreated. Practitioners need to consider how they obtain the correct information to ascertain the presence or absence of such conditions. For people with specific conditions there are often further health issues relating to their specific condition, which are well documented (Emerson, 2009; Mansell, 2010) yet are often not addressed. People with Down's syndrome, for example, may not receive regular thyroid screening despite higher frequencies of hypo-thyroidism than in the general population. In addition, they will commonly experience overproduction of earwax, dermatitis, and more serious problems such as breast lumps or major cardiac arrhythmias (Prasher, 2004). Practitioners need to apply advanced assessment skills to provide an effective and acceptable response to meet such needs. It can be daunting to face an individual with a novel symptom and a complex clinical history, who also has significant, additional communication difficulties. Development of specialist skills to meet such needs or drawing on those of others is a rewarding approach.

Clinical competencies

In addition to the required organisational changes and reasonable adjustments, clear competencies are needed to ensure appropriate interventions occur. Individual practitioners or teams may choose to develop specific competencies, for example in epilepsy, Down's syndrome or other co-morbidities, to enhance their skills.

Defining specialist input

Practitioners should know when the needs presented by people with learning disabilities are beyond their competencies. This is particularly important for conditions such as epilepsy – a very high level of seizures may be accepted when in fact specialist referral is necessary.

Communication and consent

Issues of communication and consent need to be attended to. For example, pictures can enable a person to understand something he/she may not have been able to understand previously, thus making them capable of making the decision in question (Wong et al., 2000).

> **Reflection Point 36**
>
> Try describing your job and the reason you like it using words of only four letters or less.
>
> How easy is it?
>
> What feelings does it evoke? (Frustration? Confusion? Irritation?)
>
> How much more time did it take than using your usual vocabulary?
>
> Think about the implications for your professional practice with people with learning disabilities. What challenges do you think you face in presenting easy to understand information which promotes informed choices?

Judgements and decision making

Working with people with learning disabilities in health or social care is characterised by a complex of practical and contextual factors such as:

- heterogeneity of the population
- the diversity of practice
- the emphasis on individualisation
- multiple staff roles
- unpredictable life circumstances.

All professionals make judgements under conditions of uncertainty. This can be particularly true when faced with an individual with a learning disability who may not 'fit' the usual pattern that practitioners are familiar with. Decision research has shown that in such uncertain situations, individuals do not always act rationally, coherently, or in a way that fully utilises their resources (Garfield and Garfield, 2000). Clinical guidelines, eligibility criteria and pathways are increasingly common in health and social care settings. Their purpose is to eliminate some of the cognitive biases that practitioners may introduce into the decision-making process in an attempt to reduce its uncertainty. There are some important considerations about their application in practice, for example that implementation of guidelines is slow and they may be implemented selectively. Clinical guidelines are often based on randomised trials that do not always reflect the complexity of the real world, in which a decision's context and framework are important, highlighting the difficulties in applying general guidelines. Practitioners may be more willing to use guidelines in making those judgements if research can demonstrate the guidelines' effectiveness in improving decision making for individual patients (Garfield and Garfield, 2000).

Burton and Chapman (2004) discuss how most practitioners have their own way of understanding the relationships between different situations and contexts, with different participants, different practices, and different outcomes. Practitioners' own practical theories help contextualise and clarify the often chaotic and conflicting realities by 'filling in the gaps'. Research evidence can refine and articulate links in theory, or suggest an alternative view, but gaps will exist. Evidence that does not engage with these practical theories is likely to have little impact on practice, and hence on outcomes. It is, therefore, essential that practitioners feel confident to draw on elements of their own practice (practice based evidence) such as

- experience
- appraisal of current situation
- values, attitudes, beliefs
- theory, which has several levels of explicitness
- knowledge, from multiple sources (personal, scientific, local, interpersonal, feedback from people receiving the service)
- imperatives, motivations and drivers (personal, interpersonal, organisational, professional, legal, government policy)
- judgement.

Trede and Higgs (2003) discuss how many practitioners are moving away from claiming an expert role and becoming increasingly collaborative in the decision-making processes, changing the power dynamic. Collaborative practitioners tend not to rely solely on an objective scientific view of evidence based practice but evaluate the cultural and political influences with regard to what counts as evidence. This is resulting in critical self-reflection, questioning taken-for-granted practice and the transformation of current practice. Trede and Higgs (2003) suggest this is leading to more realistic and appropriate approaches to decision making, leading to sustainable outcomes and increased patient and practitioner satisfaction. This requires practitioners to re-think their practice knowledge and the power balance of practitioner relationships with those they provide a service to (Trede and Higgs, 2003).

Consent

For collaborative decision-making approaches to be used effectively a good understanding of capacity and consent issues is required. Every adult, including everyone with a learning disability, must be presumed to have the mental capacity to consent or refuse treatment, unless they are:

- unable to take in or retain information provided about their treatment or care
- unable to understand the information provided
- unable to weigh up the information as part of the decision-making process (Mental Capacity Act, 2005a).

The way information is communicated to individuals with learning disabilities is a major consideration for practitioners. The importance of this is notable in its presence in the various codes of conduct; the NMC Code states that it is essential that nurses and midwives ensure that they:

> share with people, in a way they can understand, the information they want or need to know about their health. [And further that] you must make arrangements to meet people's language and communication needs. [And be] aware of the legislation regarding mental capacity, ensuring that people who lack capacity remain at the centre of decision making and are fully safeguarded. (NMC, 2008: 2)

The Mental Capacity Act (2005b) also requires practitioners to take into account, so far as is reasonable and practicable, the views of the patient's nearest relative and their carer.

Ethics

The paradigms of professional codes of conduct, ideas of decision making and collaboration, and legislative requirements such as the Mental Capacity Act of 2005 combine to provide practitioners with a sound ethical framework to guide approaches and decisions in their work with people with learning disabilities. Underpinning such a framework are the four principles of:

Beneficence – the obligation to provide benefits and to balance benefits against risks

Non-maleficence – the obligation to avoid causing harm

Respect for autonomy – the obligation to respect the decision-making capacities of autonomous people

Justice – the obligation of fairness, in the distribution of benefits and risks. (Gillon, 1994: 1152)

Practitioners will inevitably face ethical dilemmas from either their direct work, or arising from choices made by people with learning disabilities. There will undoubtedly be differences in the availability of support for practitioners, such as policies and procedures or training which can help to guide approaches. In line with the move towards collaborative approaches to decision making, types of additional support are reflective and sharing opportunities; this can include talking to colleagues, reflective practice, multidisciplinary working, clinical supervision, access to evidence bases, and training (Holloway, 2004).

The ethical, regulatory and policy frameworks to which practitioners are accountable, their personal desire to improve the lives of people with learning disabilities, and the relational aspects of such work can raise strong feelings that can at times feel intolerable and at other times richly rewarding. Being in a professional relationship with a person with a learning disability is central to improving their quality of life; therefore, the relational as well as procedural aspects of professional support need to be considered. Without due consideration and acknowledgement there is a risk of dehumanising both practitioners and individuals by neglecting what is core to such work, that is, the privilege of being with unique others, bearing witness to their histories and supporting them to live their lives (Wilson et al., 2009).

Confidentiality

Adults with learning disabilities, like all adults, have the right to absolute confidentiality, unless there is concern about abuse or risk of abuse. Confidential information is given in trust or obtained by a practitioner in the course of carrying out their responsibilities. When a practitioner is given this information they are obliged to keep it confidential. It is important that people with a learning disability are involved or consulted in decisions that have the effect of disclosing confidential information about them. The three areas of law that deal with confidentiality are:

- common law
- Human Rights Act (1998)
- Data Protection Act (1998).

The Data Protection Act (1998) covers all social services and health records. The Act says that access to information can be given if it is deemed in the person's best interest, for example in the case of alleged abuse or neglect or the risk of abuse and neglect. Giving access to information in these circumstances is called 'disclosure'. The Act does not prevent information being collected or disclosed; instead, it takes appropriate measures to restrict unauthorised access to personal information. Personal information can be disclosed to a third party, such as a parent, if it is necessary to protect the best interests of the individual. This would apply to someone with a learning disability who lacks mental capacity to consent to disclosure.

People with a learning disability may not have as much control over confidential information as people without a learning disability. They may have difficulty in speaking up for themselves, making them less independent and self-reliant. There are often many people involved in their lives which can make confidentiality difficult. This means confidential information often has to be shared on a 'need to know' basis with other team members. Issues around confidentiality should neither be used as a reason for not listening to carers, nor for not discussing fully with individuals the need for carers to receive information to facilitate continued support. Carers should be given sufficient information, in a way they can understand, to help them provide care efficiently.

The following points will help practitioners ensure that outcomes for people with learning disabilities, in terms of their confidentiality, are in line with those of the general population:

- ensure each person with learning disabilities is aware of their right to confidentiality
- inform each person with learning disabilities that their privacy will be respected at all times
- agree clear boundaries to confidentiality with each person, ensuring they are aware of who has access to their information and which events would impede their right to confidentiality
- work towards building an appropriate relationship with each person so that they feel confident to share information
- refer concerns/anxieties/disclosure of abuse to the relevant agency, while making sure each person is aware of the process
- be familiar with guidelines on legal constraints to maintaining confidentiality
- inform people with learning disabilities about complaints policies and procedures and support them to use these as appropriate. (Littlejohn et al., 2004)

CONCLUSION

This chapter has explored the concept of professionalism and identified the key aspects of professional practice in working with learning disabled people. The background and policy context has been discussed, with practitioners' responsibilities for bringing about real inclusion of people with learning disabilities being clearly identified. The key themes from professional codes of conduct have been identified, codes which provide a useful and familiar framework to guide practitioners through the complexities of providing meaningful and inclusive professional care to people with learning disabilities. A clear emphasis arises from both the policy context and codes of conduct on the importance of placing learning disabled people and their quality of life at the centre of professional approaches. This includes sharing power and decision making, respecting confidentiality, and ensuring that professional judgements are based on sound ethical principles and considered and transparent values. The benefits of having such approaches firmly embedded in everyday practices extend beyond individuals with learning disabilities and individual practitioners themselves, embracing cultural shifts in all spheres of professional practice and the communities in which it is delivered. Such shifts represent the future shape of service delivery in which practitioners and those they provide services to, work in partnership for effective care.

🔑 Key Learning Points 🔑

- Professionalism requires attention to beliefs, attitudes and behaviours. Beliefs are the causes of our attitudes, which in turn cause our behaviours
- A social model of disability is an appropriate framework for delivering modern professional practice
- Codes of practice share common elements across health and social care professions, creating a positive framework to deliver appropriate services to people with learning disabilities
- The health and social care needs of people with learning disabilities can and should be met through mainstream services with reasonable adjustment as required. Specialist skills should be drawn on to facilitate this or to provide additional support as and when required
- People with learning disabilities and their carers should be included in decision-making and given the appropriate support to do so with due regard to their rights to confidentiality.

REFERENCES

Benton, D.C. (1997) 'Networking', *Nursing Standard,* 35: 47–52.

Bernal, C. (2005) 'Maintenance of oral health in people with learning disabilities', *Nursing Times,* 101 (6): 40–42.

Burton, M. and Chapman, M. (2004) 'Problems of evidence based practice in community based services', *Journal of Learning Disabilities,* 8: 56–70.

Data Protection Act (1998) London: HMSO.

Department of Health (2002) *Code of Conduct for NHS Managers.* [online] Available from http://www.dh.gov.uk/en/Publicationsandstatistics/Publications/Publications PolicyAndGuidance/DH_4005410, accessed 18.03.2011.

Department of Health (2008) *Secretary of State for Health Report on Disability Equality.* London: Department of Health.

Disability Discrimination Act (1995 amended 2006) London: HMSO.

Downie, R.S. (1990) 'Professions and professionalism', cited in D. Morrell (2003) 'What is professionalism?', *Catholic Medical Quarterly*. [online] Available from http://www.catholicdoctors.org.uk/index.htm, accessed 05.04.2011.

Duggan, M., Cooper, A. and Foster, J. (2002) *Modernising the Social Model in Mental Health: A Discussion Paper*. Leeds: TOPSS/Social Perspectives Network.

Emerson, E. (2009) *Estimating Future Numbers of Adults with PMLD in England*. Lancaster: Lancaster University Centre for Disability Research.

Emerson, E. and Baines S. (2010) *Health Inequalities and People with Learning Disabilities in the UK: 2010 Improving Health and Lives Learning Disability Observatory*. [online] Available from http://www.improvinghealthandlives.org.uk/uploads/doc/vid_7479_IHaL2010-3HealthInequality2010.pdf, accessed 27.06.2011.

Equality Act (2010) London: HMSO.

Garfield, F.B. and Garfield, J.M. (2000) 'Clinical judgment and clinical practice guidelines', *International Journal of Technology Assessment in Health Care*, 16: 1050–60.

General Social Care Council (GSCC) (2010) *Codes of Practice for Social Care Workers*. London: General Social Care Council.

Gillon, R. (1994) *Principles of Health Care Ethics*. Chichester: Wiley-Blackwell

Health Professions Council (HPC) (2008) *Standards of Conduct, Performance and Ethics*. London: Health Professions Council.

Holloway, D. (2004) 'Ethical dilemmas in community learning disabilities nursing. What helps nurses resolve ethical dilemmas that result from choices made by people with learning disabilities?', *Journal of Learning Disabilities*, 8 (3): 283–98.

Howarth, A. (ed.) (2006) *Network Briefing. Key Lessons for Network Management in Health*. London: National Coordinating Centre for the Service Delivery and Organisation. London School of Hygiene and Tropical Medicine.

Human Rights Act (1998) London: HMSO.

Hunter, S. and Kendrick, M. (2009) 'The ambiguities of professional and societal wisdom', *Ethics and Social Welfare*, 3 (2): 158–69.

Junki, K. (2006) 'Networks, network governance and networked networks', *International Review of Public Administration*, 11 (1): 19–34.

Klotz, J. (2004) 'Socio cultural study of intellectual disability: moving beyond labelling and social constructionist perspectives', *British Journal of Learning Disabilities*, 32: 93–4.

Littlejohn, A., Mason, A., Schaffer, C., Reid, G., Kellock, J., Mathieson, J., Green, L., Wright, P. and Yates, R. (2004) *Making Choices Keeping Safe*. [online] Available from http://www.mcks.scot.nhs.uk/section1/1_2.html, accessed 06.04.2011.

Mansell, J. (2010) *Raising Our Sights: Services for Adults with Profound Intellectual and Multiple Disabilities*. London: HMSO.

Mencap (2007) *Death by Indifference*. London: Mencap.

Mental Capacity Act (2005a) Mental Capacity Act 2005. London: HMSO.

Mental Capacity Act (2005b) Mental Capacity Act 2005 (Transitional and Consequential Provisions) Order 2007. London: HMSO. [online] Available from http://www.legislation.gov.uk/uksi/2007/1898/contents/made, accessed on 28.03.2011.

Michael Report (2008) *Healthcare for All: Report of the Independent Inquiry into access to Healthcare for People with Learning Disabilities*. London: Department of Health.

Morrell, D. (2003) 'What is professionalism?', *Catholic Medical Quarterly*. [online] Available from http://www.catholicdoctors.org.uk/index.htm, accessed 05.04.2011.

Murphy, G. (2009) 'Challenging behaviour: a barrier to inclusion?', *Journal of Policy and Practice in Intellectual Disabilities*, 6 (2): 89–90.

Nursing and Midwifery Council (NMC) (2008) *The Code*. London: Nursing and Midwifery Council.

Office of Disability Issues (2010) *The Social Model of Disability*. [online] Available from http://odi.dwp.gov.uk/about-the-odi/the-social-model.php, accessed 06.04.2011.

Parliamentary and Health Service Ombudsman (2009) *Six Lives: The Provision of Public Services to People with Learning Disabilities*. London: HMSO.

Pawlyn, J. and Carnaby, S (eds) (2009) *Profound Intellectual and Multiple Disabilities: Nursing Complex Needs*. Oxford: Wiley-Blackwell.

Prasher, V. (2004) *Down's Syndrome and Health Care*. Kidderminster: British Institute of Learning Disabilities.

Royal College of Nursing (2008) *Dignity in Health Care for People with Learning Disabilities*. London: Royal College of Nursing.

Royal College of Nursing (RCN) (2011) *Learning Disabilities*. [online] Available from http://www.rcn.org.uk/development/practice/social_inclusion/learning_disabilities, accessed 05.04.2011.

Trede, F. and Higgs, J. (2003) 'Re-framing the clinician's role in collaborative clinical decision making: re-thinking practice knowledge and the notion of clinician–patient relationships', *Learning in Health and Social Care*, 2 (2): 66–73.

Wilson, N., Meininger, H.P. and Charnock, D. (2009) 'The agony and the inspiration: professionals' account of working with people with learning disabilities', *Mental Health Review Journal*, 14 (2): 4–13.

Wong, J.G., Clare, I.C.H., Holland, A.J., Watson, P.C. and Gunn, M.J. (2000) 'The capacity of people with a "mental disability" to make a health care decision', *Psychological Medicine*, 30 (2): 295–306.

Wullink, M., Widdershoven, G., Van Schrojenstein Lantman-de-Valk, H., Metsemakers, J. and Dinant, G. (2009) 'Autonomy in relation to health among people with intellectual disability: a literature review', *Journal of Intellectual Disability Research*, 53 (9): 816–26.

INDEX